Blockchain for Healthcare Systems

Innovations in Health Informatics and Healthcare: Using Artificial Intelligence and Smart Computing

Series Editors:
Rashmi Agrawal, Manav Rachna
International Institute of Research and Studies, and Mamta Mittal,
G.B. Pant Government Engineering College

The aim of this series is to publish reference books and handbooks that will provide conceptual and advanced reference material centered around Health Informatics and Healthcare using AI and Smart Computing. There are numerous fields within the healthcare sector where these technologies are applicable including successful ways of handling patients during a pandemic time. Large volumes of data, data analysis, and smart computing devices like IoT for sensing health data have drastically changed the way the healthcare sector functions. The scope of the book series is to report the latest advances and developments in the field of Health Informatics with the use of the latest technologies. Each book will describe in detail the use of AI, Smart Computing, Evolutionary Computing, Deep Learning, and Data Analysis in the field of Health Informatics and the books will include real-life problems that focus on the Healthcare System.

Intelligent Computing Applications for COVID-19
Predictions, Diagnosis, and Prevention
Edited by Tanzila Saba and Amjad Rehman

Blockchain for Healthcare Systems
Challenges, Privacy, and Securing of Data
Edited by Sheikh Mohammad Idrees, Parul Agarwal, and M. Afshar Alam

For more information on this series, please visit: https://www.routledge.com/Innovations-in-Health-Informatics-and-Healthcare-Using-Artificial-Intelligence-and-Smart-Computing/book-series/CRCIHIHUAISM

Blockchain for Healthcare Systems

Challenges, Privacy, and Securing of Data

Edited by
Sheikh Mohammad Idrees,
Parul Agarwal, and M. Afshar Alam

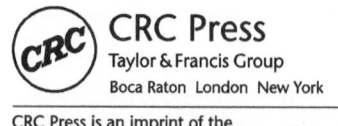

CRC Press
Taylor & Francis Group
Boca Raton London New York

CRC Press is an imprint of the
Taylor & Francis Group, an **informa** business

First edition published 2022
by CRC Press
6000 Broken Sound Parkway NW, Suite 300, Boca Raton, FL 33487-2742

and by CRC Press
2 Park Square, Milton Park, Abingdon, Oxon, OX14 4RN

Library of Congress Cataloging-in-Publication Data
Names: Idrees, Shiekh Mohammad, editor. | Agarwal, Parul, editor. |
Alam, M. Afshar, editor.
Title: Blockchain for healthcare systems : challenges, privacy, and
securing of data / edited by Shiekh Mohammad Idrees, Parul Agarwal, and
M. Afshar Alam.
Description: First edition. | Boca Raton : CRC Press, 2022. | Series:
Innovations in health informatics and healthcare: using artificial
intelligence and smart computing | Includes bibliographical references
and index.
Identifiers: LCCN 2021016379 (print) | LCCN 2021016380 (ebook) |
ISBN 9780367693527 (hardback) | ISBN 9780367693534 (paperback) |
ISBN 9781003141471 (ebook)
Subjects: LCSH: Medical records--Data processing—Security measures. |
Blockchains (Databases)
Classification: LCC R864 .B533 2022 (print) | LCC R864 (ebook) |
DDC 610.285—dc23
LC record available at https://lccn.loc.gov/2021016379
LC ebook record available at https://lccn.loc.gov/2021016380

ISBN: 978-0-367-69352-7 (hbk)
ISBN: 978-0-367-69353-4 (pbk)
ISBN: 978-1-003-14147-1 (ebk)

DOI: 10.1201/9781003141471

Typeset in Times
by codeMantra

This book is dedicated to:

Janab Hakeem Abdul Hameed

(Founder Jamia Hamdard)
(14th Sept. 1908 – 22 July 1999)

Contents

Foreword

It gives me immense pleasure to write the Foreword for the editors Sheikh Mohammad Idrees, Parul Agarwal and M. Afshar Alam. The title of the book *Blockchain for Healthcare Systems: Challenges, Privacy, and Securing of Data* looks appealing and is very relevant in today's COVID-19 pandemic-challenged world.

The book is organized into 13 chapters and is a journey from the basics to applications of blockchain in healthcare while exploring its limitations and solutions. The technology is still in its infancy, making this book covering its various aspects very handy. The blockchain system creates a decentralized, shared ledger and has an advantage in ensuring the security and privacy of data. The first chapter identifies blockchain as an intangible strategic resource whose potential needs to be exploited in today's era, a technology-driven economy. The next few chapters lay stress on applications of blockchain in the healthcare industry. The data generated from healthcare sector is massive in nature. Blockchain can have a plethora of use-cases ranging from safe management of patients' records and clinical reports to handling interoperability. Providing feedback, drug traceability, handling clinical trials, transparent insurance related contracts, automation of claims and bills, and patient data management in a secure manner (using public-key cryptography) are some of the other avenues in which it can prove to be effective. COVID-19 has unfortunately gripped the entire world. A better healthcare supply chain management was recognized as the need of the hour in this pandemic. Blockchain's solutions in drug and vaccines traceability and its delivery across states and international boundaries to tackle a situation like this pandemic are discussed. Later chapters focus on the challenges associated with blockchain's adoption and implementation at a larger scale and its downsides. The legal and regulatory aspects related to blockchain are yet to be explored. The last chapter discusses blockchain's acceptability in developing jurisdictions and deliberations in the context of India.

A worthy read, the book would serve as one of the prominent resources highlighting blockchain for healthcare in a clear and concise manner. Much recommended!

Prof. M.N. Doja,
Director, IIIT Sonepat

Preface

Blockchain is more than just a novel decentralized technology. It is also an emerging technology that disrupts and revolutionizes many sectors of our society, in the financial sector, industry and institutions. Blockchain and decentralization can help to solve many of industry's challenges, among others, interoperability. Blockchain technology is going to revolutionize all sectors of human life apart from just finance and crypto-currency. Various sectors are reshaped by the new trusted data models enabled and inspired by blockchain – and healthcare is no exception. In fact, healthcare may hold the greatest opportunities for meaningful use of the technology. Early pioneers have explored some of the first use-cases for medical payments, electronic health records, data privacy, drug counterfeiting and credentialing of healthcare professionals. We have only begun to scratch the surface of how to address the complexities of today's healthcare systems and design new systems that focus on trust, transparency and the alignment of incentives. The healthcare sector faces several challenges associated with the handling of data and privacy and security issues of data, as blockchain is the only technology that guarantees consensus between all parties who are unwilling to trust one other. Implementation of blockchain technology in the healthcare sector will facilitate a transition from institution-driven interoperability to patient-centred interoperability.

This book lays focus on the concepts of technology and how new technologies can work in an integrated manner with existing technologies. The healthcare data and blockchain-based solutions can be identified for handling the data. The technology should be responsive to the challenges associated with healthcare and should also be able to combat them. Future directions have been explored as well. The technology is already being used to manage the outbreak of harmful diseases. In particular, blockchain-based approaches for COVID-19 can also be dealt with. The decentralized nature of ledger-based technology allows the stakeholders, namely doctors, patients and healthcare providers, to share information quickly (providing transparency), besides concealing identity and thus handling sensitive data. These make the technology rife with several security applications. This book facilitates sharing of both theoretical and practical knowledge required for blockchain approaches for healthcare and highlights the state of the art in their development.

This book is intended for healthcare professionals, researchers, academicians and students who seek to gain an insight into the concepts and applications of blockchain technology with respect to healthcare, particularly with respect to the security and privacy aspects.

BOOK CONTENTS

This book comprises 13 chapters, designed to capture the core ideas of blockchain and healthcare, and is organized as follows:

Chapter 1: Blockchain Technology: A Strategic Resource

Blockchain has indeed been realized and utilized as a strategic resource. This chapter offers literature and discusses its applications and identifies its potential to prove the same. Its utilization and growing importance need to be identified in the modern era. Additionally, with respect to healthcare, there is a need for keeping in mind the measures required for attaining a sustained advantage.

Chapter 2: Blockchain Technology and Its Applications in the Healthcare Sector

Bitcoin implementation has expedited the technological innovation in the form of blockchain technology. Blockchain, we all realize, has a significant impact on healthcare. Traditional health practices are changing due to the adoption of this technology. This chapter highlights the applications and developments being brought about in the healthcare sector because of blockchain. Blockchain has to be seen in the light of its future perspectives and challenges that it faces. This chapter explores these in detail.

Chapter 3: An Overview of Blockchain Technology Concepts from a Modern Perspective

Blockchain, a shared digital ledger, contains all information related to a transaction and is accessible to all its participating users. This chapter throws light on blockchain and its usage in healthcare with a modern outlook to it. Today, things have revolutionized. The challenges associated with traditional practices including maintaining electronic health records, sharing information for global diseases worldwide, data record management, security and privacy issues related to the records of personal data and clinical reports, etc. have been truly overcome by blockchain. This chapter effectively evaluates the same.

Chapter 4: Blockchain Technology: A Panacea for Medical Distribution Ailments

The times change, and certain things come as an awakening in our lives. During these unprecedented times, when COVID-19 has gripped the entire world, it also awakened our minds and blockchain technology has come as a great help in providing relief to the healthcare sector. In earlier times, when availability of medicines and their delivery across borders (national and international), during such tough times were a weak possibility, blockchain, on the other hand, had combated it effectively. The management of the health supply chain during such times was the need of the hour. The health supply chain faces several logistical complexities: lack of visibility into shipment and goods tracing, quality of medical goods, transportation-related problems and fraud associated with payments. Blockchain provides transparency and usability in effective supply chain management while its shortcomings are also explored.

Chapter 5: Digital Transformation in Healthcare: Innovation and Technologies

Medical care, better clinical trials, better data management and storage, transparency in the reports, sharing of medical records among stakeholders with different level of access, etc. are some of the benefits that blockchain provides. This chapter not only looks at healthcare with blockchain perspectives, but also explores various innovations that are taking place because of blockchain. Not just implementing innovations but also adopting best approaches and practices and utilizing the benefits that blockchain provides in an effective manner are necessary. Amalgamation of various technologies and their advantages shall improve healthcare services. Artificial intelligence, augmented reality, cloud computing, big data and IoT are some of these technologies that shall aid in remote patient monitoring, diagnosis and cure, drug discovery and better healthcare services. This chapter digs into these aspects related to healthcare.

Chapter 6: Modernizing the Health Insurance Industry Using Blockchain and Smart Contracts

The Indian health insurance industry has grown substantially and is speculated to permeate each and every household. However, the insurance sector is gripped with problems: data management, security and privacy, fraud management, lack of transparency in contracts, fraud in policies and lack of shared data among various stakeholders of the industry. Blockchain can effectively combat these challenges, as it is a shared and digital ledger. In lieu of this fact, blockchain can automate these processes and provide solutions that can be harnessed effectively to improve the user experience and ease the insurance process. This chapter discusses the same and provides solutions for the above problems.

Chapter 7: Blockchain Technology Applications for Improving Quality of Electronic Healthcare System

Blockchain technology offers abundant benefits in the healthcare sector, primarily: managing health records effectively, providing secure data, ensuring privacy of details, medical supply chain management and many others. Yet, simultaneously, the quality should not be compromised for any of these applications. Besides, realizing the potential of blockchain, AI, cloud computing, machine learning and IoT for ensuring quality in healthcare goods and services is equally important. An insight into these aspects is provided by this chapter.

Chapter 8: Computing Techniques for Securing Healthcare Data with Blockchain Technology

Sharing or leakage of medical data, either personal or clinical reports, remains a major concern for the stakeholders of the healthcare sector. As COVID-19 grips us all, we know that diagnosis and treatment-related data are being shared among hospitals and other agencies involved. Thus, breach of data occurs. An inappropriate access to data becomes inevitable. To prevent this, cloud computing can provide solutions against such threats. Cloud computing provides services including: data as a service (DAAS), software as a service (SAAS), platform as a service (PAAS) and infrastructure as a service (IAAS). These services allow secured storage and patient's data analysis. In this chapter, security-enhanced machine learning blockchain (SeMB) model is proposed, with its applications in the healthcare sector while exploring its pros and cons. This model will aid in maintaining secure electronic healthcare data in health care centres.

Chapter 9: Blockchain-based Solutions for COVID-19: Challenges, Advantages and Applications

When the entire world is gripped by COVID-19, the need for upgraded healthcare services is urgent. Researchers, academicians and healthcare professionals are looking for effective solutions, particularly with respect to blockchain. This chapter focuses on opportunities that blockchain offers for the improvement of health services. Challenges associated with healthcare (pandemics in particular), solutions, and applications of the technology specifically with regard to COVID-19 are discussed. Promising use-cases for this technology in healthcare are also covered.

Chapter 10: Managing Medical Supply Chain Using Blockchain Technology

The delivery of medical goods and services in a timely and safe manner remains a critical issue in the healthcare sector. Traditional practices are unable to ensure the same. However, blockchain can help. To achieve competence and to optimize the components of the business cycle, a transparent and efficient supply chain is essential. Fake medicines, poor inventory management, loss of drug traceability en-route and delay in delivery of medical goods are the major challenges associated with supply chain management. Blockchain overcomes all these challenges and provides solutions for each of these. This chapter explores all of these aspects.

Chapter 11: Sustainable and Effective Blockchain-based Solutions for the Security and Privacy of Healthcare Data

Smart healthcare uses actuators and sensors for collecting data. This data proves effective in diagnosis, treatment and cure. In recent times, the next frontier in the healthcare system is blockchain technology though AI and smart computing techniques, which are also major technologies that play a key role in smart healthcare. It becomes crucial in today's scenario to provide sustainable and effective blockchain-based solutions which ensure a secure and private network and data management. This chapter explores these aspects in detail.

Chapter 12: Security and Privacy Concerns for Blockchain While Handling Healthcare Data

Electronic health record (EHR) refers to patient's medical records that are maintained and stored. While security and privacy are a major concern, the storage of data on cloud makes it vulnerable to even more threats. Blockchain technology is a saviour indeed. This chapter evaluates several opportunities and challenges associated with blockchain and E-health systems.

Chapter 13: Blockchain Technology in Medical Data Management and Protection in India: The Law in the Making

Blockchain technology has improved the healthcare sector substantially and shall revolutionize it in a few years. Though several challenges still confront it, its acceptability in various developing jurisdictions including that of India is to be explored.

This chapter proposes to unravel the legal position of healthcare data management and the use of technology in India to estimate the viability of blockchain technology in healthcare in the coming years. The chapter unfolds several aspects of blockchain with respect to regulations and in the domain of law. This chapter proposes a policy that may act as a guideline for the use of technology in the healthcare sector in India and also in the Global South.

I hope you delve deeper into the varied aspects of this book and enjoy reading and learning about blockchain technology with respect to healthcare. This book would not be possible without the involvement of many people. We owe our gratitude and dedicate it to our family members without whose support this wouldn't be achieved. Much appreciation goes to our authors and we are much obliged to the reviewers for their comments which improved the quality of the book. Last but not the least, thanks to God, for showing us the light to start this project and blessing us to complete it.

Sheikh Mohammed Idrees
Parul Agarwal
M. Afshar Alam

Editors

Sheikh Mohammad Idrees, PhD, earned his PhD from the Department of Computer Science, Jamia Hamdard, New Delhi. He is currently working as a postdoctoral fellow at Department of Computer Science (IDI), Norwegian University and Science and Technology. He is the recipient of Alain Bensoussan Fellowship Award under European Research Consortium for Informatics and Mathematics, Sophia Antipolis Cedex, France. He has authored or co-authored several scientific publications in well-reputed journals and international conferences. He is also a frequent book editor for Springer and CRC Press (Taylor & Francis Group) books apart from being a frequent reviewer of various reputed international journals and conferences.

Parul Agarwal, PhD, has been associated with Jamia Hamdard since 2002. She is currently an Associate Professor in the Department of Computer Science and Engineering. Her areas of specialization include fuzzy data mining, cloud computing, blockchain technology and soft computing. Her particular interests include sustainable computing and its applications in agriculture, transportation and healthcare. She has published several research papers in well-reputed conferences and journals indexed in SCI, ISI, Scopus and other scientific databases. She also has many book chapters published by CRC Press, Springer and IGI-Global to her credit. She has chaired several sessions of international/national conferences of high repute. Currently, she is supervising the work of several PhD scholars. Dr. Agarwal is a member of several committees at university level and several professional bodies including ISTE and IEEE.

M. Afshar Alam, PhD, earned his PhD in computer science from Jamia Millia Islamia, New Delhi. He has served as the Dean of School, DSW, and Foreign Students' Advisor with Jamia Hamdard, New Delhi, where he is a full-time Professor, head and Dean of the School of Engineering Science and Technology. He is well known internationally for his work. He is also an invited professor at various universities all over the world. Dr. Alam is also an expert member of various government committees in India. He has more than 24 years of teaching experience and has supervised more than 25 PhD students in all these years. He has published more than 130 research articles in well-reputed journals, besides authoring several books. His research interests include the areas of data analytics, cloud computing, big data, applied machine learning, predictive modeling, AI, sustainable development, cybersecurity and time series analysis.

Contributors

Ali Akbar
Department of Computer Science
  and Engineering
Jamia Hamdard
New Delhi, India

Mohammad Amjad
Department of Computer Engineering
  Faculty of Engineering &
  Technology
Jamia Millia Islamia
New Delhi, India

Kumari Anjali
School of Management Studies (SOMS)
IGNOU
New Delhi, India

Rangel Arthur
School of Technology (FT)
State University of Campinas
  (UNICAMP)
Limeira, São Paulo, Brazil

Mohd Adnan Baig
Department of Computer Science
  and Engineering
Jamia Hamdard
New Delhi, India

Pankaj Bhatt
School of Pharmacy
Glocal University
Saharanpur, India

Shambhu Prasad Chakrabarty
Centre for Regulatory Studies,
  Governance and Public
  Policy
The West Bengal National University
  of Juridical Sciences
Kolkata, West Bengal

Richa Chauhan
Department of Commerce &
  Management
Banasthali Vidyapith
Rajasthan, India

Anubha Dubey
Independent researcher
  and analyst
Noida, India

Reinaldo Padilha França
School of Electrical Engineering
  and Computing (FEEC)
State University of Campinas
  (UNICAMP)
Campinas, São Paulo, Brazil

Pooja Gupta
Department of Computer Science
  and Engineering
Jamia Hamdard
New Delhi, India

Yuzo Iano
School of Electrical Engineering and
  Computing (FEEC)
State University of Campinas
  (UNICAMP)
Campinas, São Paulo, Brazil

Sheikh Mohammad Idrees
Department of Computer Science (IDI)
Norwegian University of Science
  and Technology
Gjøvik, Norway

Zubair Jeelani
Department of Computer Sciences
Islamic University of Science
  and Technology
J&K, India

Nikhil Kant
School of Management Studies (SOMS)
IGNOU
New Delhi, India

Vidhi Kaul
Independent researcher

Abdullah Mohammad Ali Khan
Department of Computer Science
    and Engineering
Jamia Hamdard
New Delhi, India

Dawood Ashraf Khan
Department of Computer Sciences
University of Kashmir
J&K, India

Ihtiram Raza Khan
Department of Computer Science
    and Engineering
Jamia Hamdard
New Delhi, India

Vipin Kumar
School of Pharmacy
Glocal University
Saharanpur, India

Ana Carolina Borges Monteiro
School of Electrical Engineering
    and Computing (FEEC)
State University of Campinas
    (UNICAMP)
Campinas, São Paulo, Brazil

Souvik Mukherjee
The West Bengal National University
    of Juridical Sciences
Kolkata, West Bengal

Neha
Department of Computer Science
    and Engineering
Jamia Hamdard
New Delhi, India

S. Rabiu
School of Pharmacy
Glocal University
Saharanpur, India

Ishfaq Hussain Rather
School of Computer and Systems
    Sciences
Jawaharlal Nehru University
New Delhi, India

Satish Kumar Sharma
School of Pharmacy
Glocal University
Saharanpur, India

Suruchi Singh
School of Pharmacy
Glocal University
Saharanpur, India

Apurva Saxena Verma
Researcher computer science
Bhopal, India

Rameez Yousuf
Department of Computer Sciences
University of Kashmir
J&K, India

Sana Zeba
Department of Computer Engineering
Faculty of Engineering & Technology
    of Jamia Millia Islamia
New Delhi, India

1 Blockchain Technology
A Strategic Resource

Nikhil Kant and Kumari Anjali
IGNOU

CONTENTS

1.1 INTRODUCTION

Constant advancements and growing significance of information and communication technology (ICT) have brought about a plethora of transformations requiring organizations to rethink the viability of conventional competition and value-generation which have lost considerable strategic effectiveness. In recent times, the liberalized, privatized, and globalized world has witnessed increased competition due to the presence or emergence of abundant organizations with almost similar objectives. Technological advancements, in the current much-hyped fourth industrial revolution which has introduced multiple innovations including blockchain – a digitally distributed ledger – have made their presence felt by remarkably influencing almost all aspects of our routine lives. They have brought forward many opportunities and challenges. In the changing landscape, the healthcare system cannot remain insulated from these risks and opportunities. A World Economic Forum (WEF) survey conducted in 2015 found that government use of blockchain would peak by 2023 (Kant, 2020). While blockchain has attracted huge investments from governments and other organizations such as banks, software organizations, and stock exchanges, the fast expansion of its use beyond the financial sector indicates that the healthcare system can also look forward to using it as a strategic resource.

The omnipresent learning environments can largely be benefitted from blockchain in finding solutions to the issues of vulnerability, privacy, and security (Bdiwi et al. 2017). The idiosyncrasies of blockchain in education can be witnessed in the enhancement of the certificate management with greater digital infrastructural data security and trust (Xu et al., 2017), and digital accreditation of the learning

DOI: 10.1201/9781003141471-1

(Grech & Camilleri, 2017). Zhao et al. (2016) argue in favor of the increasing relevance of blockchain which gets support from IBM Corp. (2016). IBM Corp. (2016) informs about the declaration of more than one-third of C-suite executives as regards their consideration to engage with or already active engagement with blockchain. Christidis and Devetsikiotis (2016) posit that developers and researchers have already acquainted themselves with its huge capabilities and explored different applications in different sectors.

Blockchain, an open-source resource, has commonly been known as the core technology behind cryptocurrencies and has a very short history of merely a decade. In this short period, it has demonstrated its potential with a number of applications being used commercially in different industries sparking increasing interest from various industries and academic institutions in Europe and other countries (Grech and Camilleri 2017). This scenario hints at the need to explore its potential of revolutionizing the healthcare system also. Organizations creating the healthcare system desire and make commensurate effort to attain and sustain competitive advantage harnessing their capabilities of combining internal and external tangible and intangible resources for converting them into idiosyncratic for strategic utilization. With the fast adoption of digitization, healthcare has accumulated huge patients' records in electronic form demanding greater security in using and exchanging these data where blockchain offers huge potentials as a responsible and transparent data distributing and storage mechanism, providing solutions to serious challenges related to data security, privacy, and integrity in healthcare (Khezr et al., 2019; Yaeger et al., 2019). Blockchain being a disruptive technological innovation has been encouraging the healthcare system to take appropriate strategic steps for achieving competitiveness and sustaining it further.

Literature shows consensus in considering contributions of innovations in the creation of competitiveness, and in recent past, the focus has increased on technological innovations (Weerawardena & Mavondo, 2011) with the supporting arguments that intangible resources, which include technological innovations also, are more strategic than tangible resources (Barney, 1991; Hitt et al., 2001). However, strategic use of blockchain in healthcare system either as the best-fitted technology or as an innovation is yet to be assessed, considering that an invention with successful commercial utility only can be construed as an innovation (Kant, 2020). For this, organizations in healthcare sector must apply blockchain-enabled applications for effective decision-making in order to bridge the chasm between expectations, priorities, practices, and models making use of their updated strategic informational knowledge of the dynamic developments and anticipated future trends.

Casino et al. (2019), in a comprehensive systematic review, have argued that limited attention has been paid to the state-of-the-art blockchain-enabled applications. This is despite several reviews focusing on its specific role in developing data-intensive applications and managing big data in a decentralized fashion, potential to enable trust and decentralization in service system, its security issues and technical aspects of its design, usability, data integrity, scalability, currency aspect, and security and privacy. Blockchain offers the huge potential to create competitiveness. Healthcare system can be one among multiple probable beneficiaries expecting useful disruptions with the support of idiosyncratic characteristics including but not limited to decentralization, traceability, immutability, reliability, trustworthiness, self-sovereignty, currency properties, transparency, provenance, disintermediation, collaboration, security, efficiency, etc. (Kant, 2020).

While the healthcare system is yet to taste the benefits offered by blockchain, the issue of considering it as a strategic resource for healthcare system faces inadequacy of relevant literature. However, in recent times, there has been a remarkable generation of interest among academics and industries toward blockchain with blockchain-enabled applications, and relevant research is coming up with new solutions almost every day (Khezr et al., 2019; Yaeger et al., 2019). With multiple applications in healthcare, blockchain offers potentialities for the improvement of monitoring devices, mobile health applications, and exchange and storage of electronic medical records, clinical trial information, insurance information. Despite the limitations of research studies, blockchain is set to transform the healthcare system with the support of its decentralized principles, thereby improving secured accessibility of patient information, changing the healthcare hierarchy, and developing a new patient-managed system of their own care (Chen et al., 2019). This chapter seeks to discuss blockchain as a strategic resource that can help healthcare system attain and sustain competitive advantage with the increased applications volume, and heightens significance for researchers, professionals, and policymakers.

1.2   KNOWING ABOUT BLOCKCHAIN

Blockchain denotes a secured information storing and sharing system with huge transparency where every block of the chain is not only its own independent unit with its own information but also a dependent link in the entire chain at the same time where a participant-regulated network is created by this duality which, without any intervention of a third party, store and share the information (Chen et al., 2019). Blockchain has gained so much popularity in recent times that on daily basis, we hear news about its new and innovative applications with the perceived disrupting ability affecting our routine daily life significantly. Blockchain is being considered as one of the most important technological trends in this century, which not only can handle big data in a secured transparent mechanism but also can lead us toward a decentralized computing future with enhanced trust and transparency significantly where common public can benefit immensely from the reduced influence of the few select powerful computing stalwarts.

Kant (2020) finds its distributed and decentralized nature and the idiosyncratic features of record permanence and smart contracts as the primary reasons behind huge perceived expectations. Hou (2017) emphasizes that applications enabled by blockchain, with the help of its idiosyncrasies in disintermediation of transactions and record keeping, offer huge potentialities in transforming the way local governments operate. He receives support from Casino et al. (2019), who favor the aims of blockchain governance in offering the same services (legal documents registration, attestation, identification, marriage contracts, taxes, voting, etc.) offered by the state and its corresponding public authorities more efficiently but maintaining the same validity in a decentralized mechanism.

Figure 1.1 provides a basic idea of how blockchain operates. Grech and Camilleri (2017) define it as a distributed digital information recording ledger, shareable in

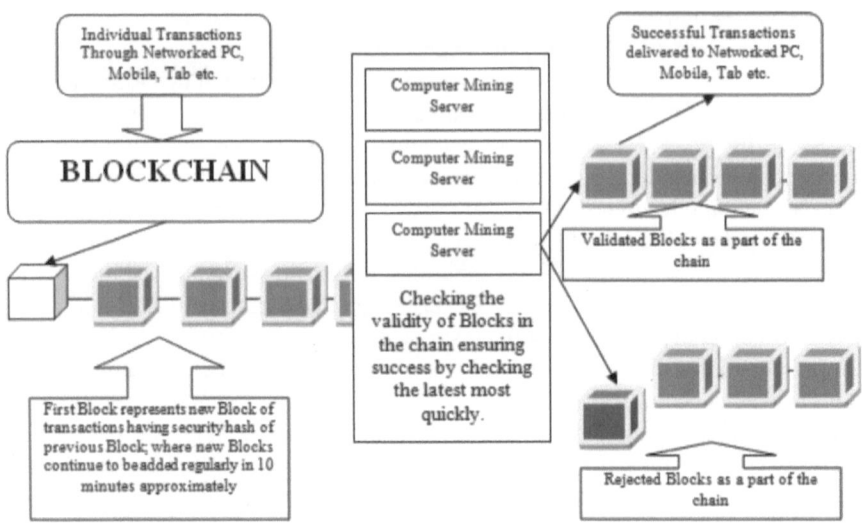

FIGURE 1.1   How blockchain operates: An overview.

a community where members maintain own data collectively validated by all the members. Members can see entire transactions history because of their permanence, transparency, and searchability. They further note that update is added to the tail of the "chain" constituting a "block" containing entries and edits which are initiated-validated-recorded-distributed by a cryptology-based protocol eliminating the need of any intermediary. It performs as the trust-keeper which, for the purpose of ensuring integrity of the system, asks participants to run complex algorithms. Blockchain is broadly referred to as "digitally distributed ledger" as it denotes a form of digital ledger to record transactions being copied to every networked computer. Blockchain is found to have idiosyncratic characteristic of keeping all the data time-stamped while the length of the chain continuously grows. Nakamoto (2008), an unknown person associated with the invention of Bitcoin, informs that blockchain uses participants-maintained distributed techniques and consensus algorithms achieved through verification mechanisms, e.g., proof-of-work. Table 1.1 illustrates the idiosyncrasies because of which blockchain may be considered strategic.

Underwood (2016) believes blockchain to be an innovative emerging technology with huge potential which, as a distributed decentralized ledger technology, acts as a shared database because of keeping all copies synced and verified. It enables members to make their own transactions in digital assets displaying distributed authority of a ledger in public domain (Nakamoto, 2008). It propagates transparency, decentralized efficient flexible reliable data management with higher security, and integrity removing any chance of centralized failure (Zhu & Zhou, 2016).

Casino et al. (2019), in a recent systematic review, differing largely from their predecessors and using a rigorous literature-based statistical methodology fitting appropriately to the current developments and future trends, found that blockchain applications have mostly been classified into financial and non-financial. They highlighted a higher representation of cryptocurrencies in the existing blockchain

TABLE 1.1

Idiosyncrasies Associated with Blockchain

IET Healthcare (2019)	Data integrity, provenance from cradle to grave, security, resilience, unalterable evidence, out of the box, no single point of failure, single source of truth, immutability, transaction history/traceability, data privacy, synchronization, dynamic consent, personal data storage clouds enabling individual access, self-executing contractual states, multilevel de-identification and encryption technologies
Chen et al. (2018)	Reliability, trust, security, efficiency, decentralization, traceability, immutability, currency properties
Grech and Camilleri (2017)	Self-sovereignty, transparency, provenance, trust, immutability, disintermediation, collaboration
Underwood (2016)	Immutability, transparency, trust

networks, or based on the blockchain versions 1.0, 2.0, and 3.0, before proposing an application-oriented classification. It is pertinent to mention what Swan (2015) has elaborated as regards its different developmental stages on a continuum starting from Blockchain 1.0 (emergence of cryptocurrencies), through Blockchain 2.0 (emergence of smart contracts in financial services and others), to the current Blockchain 3.0 (applications beyond currency, economics, and markets) with the dynamically growing list of beneficiary sectors.

Purely based on code, blockchain denotes a software solution that relies on hardware. However, arguments that "When the software is not an integral part of the related hardware, computer software is treated as an intangible asset" (Ind AS, 2015, p. 1112) suggest that it is an intangible resource as it is a software missing any centralized controlling part and exists as copies on different networked computers interconnected but not integrated with any of the hardware.

Nguyen (2016) underscores the higher expectations from blockchain in playing an essential role in achieving sustainable development of the economy and the current banking system, providing consumers and the entire society with benefits and project such as Solarcoin which might motivate for using renewable energy and therefore the use of renewable energy could be critical (Potenza, 2017). Khezr et al. (2019) highlight the huge growth in the interests of scholars and experts toward its utilization in different domains.

1.3　CHANGING LANDSCAPE OF HEALTHCARE SYSTEM

Healthcare system is under tremendous pressure to acquire and maintain greater operational efficiency, effectiveness, and sustainability in future. Its ability to optimally utilize the continuously growing health data available in conventional sources as well as electronic and digital records will be of great help in getting new insights and driving the transformation to a more patient-centric system. However, barriers restricting smooth adoption of technological innovations in healthcare system are not few and far between which include the concerns related to data consistency and quality, compatibility, security, privacy, and absence of standards (COCIR, 2017).

IET Healthcare (2019) reports that public and private healthcare sectors are facing immense pressures of the cost regulations and providing quality services to the patients. These pressures are getting more intense, day by day, with the emergence of disruptive technologies. The growing pressure needs them to search for newer cost-reducing opportunities without compromising the patient service quality. In order to live up to the expectations, their strategy needs to be aligned with these dynamic changes seeking support from the technological advancements. Blockchain offers huge potentialities to solve one of the major problems in the healthcare industry, i.e., the transmission of patient data with privacy and security, and is perceived to have a remarkable effect on health management. While the estimates of the Institute of Medicine indicate almost one-fourth of the healthcare expenditure as wasteful or a result of poor outcomes, they find high administrative fees and medical tests, useless medical treatments, missed prevention opportunities, and fraud are the main sources. Here, blockchain offers huge potentialities to enhance healthcare delivery efficiency and research opportunities by integrating or sharing data for attaining the scale desired to improve care, access, productivity, cost-efficiency, and medical breakthroughs innovations. Because of the immutable permanence of blockchain with no centralized structure for a malicious attack, blockchain can be viable and feasible in the context of healthcare data management despite its applications in healthcare are in infancy which are maturing with more and more research adding new findings every day (Chen et al., 2019).

COCIR (2017) further adds that the idiosyncratic features of blockchain make it potentially valuable for healthcare system, having a number of regularly interacting stakeholders and showing understandable excitements toward its potential. Healthcare system is expected to witness certain but gradual adoption of blockchain because of the perceived transformative potential of developing new business models.

1.4   KNOWING ABOUT STRATEGIC RESOURCE

Strategic management provides insight into how to respond to the dynamically changing conditions, exposing organizations to the changes in performance and improvement. It underlines the need to sustain competitiveness through rational and analytical competitive strategies with an advantage over competing rivals. It also underscores the need for innovations resulting from sensing opportunities and threats – seizing opportunities – and reconfiguring resources and capabilities in order to ensure prosperity in the most competitive situations as they are closely related to sustaining competitive advantages. Use of correct and recognized information can also be a strategically important resource. Using technological innovation such as blockchain, which is basically an intangible resource, therefore can be considered a strategic approach (Kant, 2020).

Competitive advantage, used as a relational term facilitating organizational comparison based on their competing abilities and competition among them, is attained by using suitable strategy of gaining positive results (Peteraf, 1993; Porter, 1980, 1985, 1990). Competitive advantage denotes an outcome of greater executing speed and agility of suitable strategy and implementing of better resources (Barney, 1991; Bharadwaj, 2000), and it (Barney, 2001) can comprise skills, methods, and capabilities of using appropriate resources optimally for outpace rivals. Barney (1991) clarifies that all the assets, capabilities, processes, attributes, information, and knowledge constitute resource which organizations by virtue of possessing get support in implementing suitable efficiency and effectiveness improving strategy. Organizations performing their different internal activities witness emergence of resources or acquire them externally which are tangible or intangible. Though both types of resources are responsible for adding economic value, intangible resources are found to be contributing strategically more that tangible resources due to the inherent attribute of inimitability (Barney, 1991; Hitt et al., 2001; Reed, 2005).

Falle et al. (2016) and Klewitz and Hansen (2014) highlight the need of appropriate decision-making for attaining competitive advantage in new markets or in the existing markets with the help of innovations. Teece et al. (1997) emphasize that the ability of combining resources effectively builds competitive advantage. As per resource-based view (RBV) theory, the attributes of resources which help in attaining sustained competitive advantage, as Barney (1991) puts it, are Value, Rareness, Inimitability, and Non-substitutability (VRIN) which organization can use to build and implement strategies for enhancing effectiveness and efficiency. Suitable efforts are made by organizations for using the resources strategically and making their attributes VRIN.

While organizations tend to attain competitive advantage with the underpinnings of the generic strategies (cost leadership, differentiation, and focus), as Porter (1980) puts it, the dynamic capabilities of integrating and reconfiguring internal and external resources, keeping in view the threats and opportunities, might be helpful for them in sustaining it responding timely to the rapid and flexible innovations (Teece, 2007; Teece and Pisano, 1994). Teece (2007) further adds the dimensions of sensing threats and opportunities, seizing them, and reconfiguring as per actual needs to sustain it.

1.5 BLOCKCHAIN: A STRATEGIC RESOURCE

Khezr et al. (2019) highlight the significant role of blockchain in professional world with its disruptive capabilities and urge to consider it to be a very important discovery in the form of chains of block covering information and maintaining trust between parties despite being much distant from one another. Casino et al. (2019) find studies focusing on the disruptive potential of blockchain in becoming a significant source of business and management innovations bringing about improvement, optimization, and automation of the processes visible through emergence of plethora of e-business models based on blockchain. These applications apparently provide remarkable enhancement of performances and commercialization opportunities (White, 2017) and save cost as well as time (IBM Corp., 2016).

Casino et al. (2019) emphasize that blockchain can be a reinforcing instrument for ensuring equality and providing opportunities to worldwide citizens citing the example of the World Citizen project used in a decentralized passport service for the purpose of identifying citizens. They further posit that virtual notary, reputation dispute resolution, among others are some of the services which require to be provided to the citizens without intermediation of the official institutions. Blockchain plays a bigger role in providing such public services in that manner. E-voting has been considered an essential development required to make the voting processes faster, simpler, and cost effective for bringing about more robust democracies, in recent times (Boucher, 2016). Potentials of blockchain as an open-source, peer-to-peer, decentralized, and independently verifiable network need to be tapped for enhancing the confidence of the voters and election organizers, argues Noizat (2015). Nakamoto (2008) reports that blockchain as a distributed peer-to-peer linked structure can provide solutions for a number of problems as regards the maintenance of the order of transactions and avoidance of double-spending.

Using technological innovation such as blockchain, which is basically an intangible resource, can be considered a strategic approach, argues Kant (2020), highlighting its strategic usefulness in attaining and sustaining competitive advantage. Casino et al. (2019) posit that the structure of blockchain manages to possess a robust and auditable registry of different transactions occurred in it which facilitates audit of these transactions. Chen et al. (2019) report that the current healthcare system has major challenges associated with data security and data ownership which need to be addressed immediately and urgently, highlighting the lack of secured structure as regards sensitive medical records causing data breaches with serious impact inability of the patients to have complete ownership of own medical data. This is an issue with increased relevance in an era of continuously growing use of personalized wearables in addition to medicine. Blockchain offers useful applications in improving mechanical security and quality of accessing and sharing of medical records, spread out across multiple healthcare facilities, resolving also the associated moral repercussions. Blockchain applied to clinical trials and medical insurance storage in recent times has favorably contributed in detecting fake information making use of transparency and security with the security promoting features of smart contracts.

COCIR (2017) reports on the basis of a number of use cases in healthcare system that blockchain provides potential opportunities which mainly include exchange of health related information, clinical trials, reimbursement of healthcare services, and supply chains. It is notable that technological advancements are responsible for the creation of plethora of business opportunities for the organizations in the healthcare system by using health data generating financial value when big data is set to play significant role in transforming the volume-based care to value-based care, also incorporating accountability. The use of blockchain offers potentialities by integrating, synthesizing, and sharing complex medical data for an improved coordination, better outcomes, and cost efficiency in the healthcare sector which is set to reap the rich harvest of greater optimization and efficiency through it (IET Healthcare, 2019).

Casino et al. (2019) and Idrees et al. (2021) find the emphasis of a number of studies highlighting the pivotal role of blockchain in the healthcare industry in their systematic review-based study taking note of its applications in areas including, but not limited to, management of public healthcare, recordkeeping of longitudinal healthcare, automated adjudications of health claims, online access and sharing of patients' medical data, user-oriented research, counterfeiting of drug, clinical trial, precision medicine, etc. Nugent et al. (2016) underscore the effective use of smart contracts integrated in the blockchain for solving multiple problems related to the scientific credibility of clinical trials' results, whereas Benchoufi and Ravaud (2017) argue in its favor for the greater usability as regards the issues of patients' informed consent. Hoy (2017) perceives immense potential growth in the field of managing Electronic Healthcare Records (EHRs) of the patients which keep their short medical history, data, predictions, and various vital pieces of information as regards their medical conditions and clinical progress during a treatment. Grey Healthcare (2017) highlighting the idiosyncrasies of a blockchain-enabled EHRs system informs its multiple benefits including, but not limited to, the storing of records in a distributed way without any centralized owner or hub restricting thereby any hacker from harming them, keeping the data updated and readily available, gathered from diverse sources in a unified data warehouse. While centralized public as well as private organizations assemble huge personal information which includes sensitive information, blockchain offers an opportunity to enhance the security aspects of such big data (Puthal et al., 2018). Extant literature, therefore, profusely encompasses privacy and security-oriented blockchain-enabled applications (Casino et al., 2019). It is notable that the resources configuration along with their utilization and utility play to be building blocks of competitive advantage for an organization (Kant, 2020; Kant & Anjali, 2020), and therefore the potentialities of blockchain in the context of healthcare system as a strategic resource need to be further explored and assessed in terms of its contributions to competitive advantage collectively with other resources and capabilities.

Deloitte (2016) highlights the potential implications of the blockchain with respect to health insurance comprising the building of a more secure data warehouse maintaining medical and wellness information in order to provide timely reminders for taking prescriptions, or diagnostic tests, making periodical visits to doctor in addition to facilitating continuous evaluation of underwriting and pricing, building more logical and updated risk pooling, and giving rise to greater personalization of the coverage. Khezr et al. (2019) highlight the dynamic growth of blockchain providing a plethora of new application opportunities which include healthcare applications also. Their study not only comprehensively reviews the emerging blockchain-enabled healthcare applications technologies and related applications but also provides a research agenda in this dynamically growing field along with an elaboration of the relevant details and the potentialities it offers to revolutionize healthcare industry.

Chen et al. (2019) point out its susceptibility to a specific 51% attack which is also known as double-spend/majority attack despite higher security integrated in blockchain, with the disclaimer that the success rate of this attack is very low, rendering one to believe blockchain to be one of the most secure technological forms. The cost of implementing blockchain is also a potential concern given the huge number of transactions to be processed in healthcare settings the impact of which can, however, be negated with the advantages associated with the replacement of existing huge storage systems and removal of costly data breaches/errors, providing the organizations cost leadership.

With the greater use of technology in healthcare system, blockchain can offer greater potentialities of revolutionizing the healthcare system. Organizations in the healthcare system endeavoring to attain competitive advantage with the appropriate use of tangible and intangible resources, in a liberalized-privatized-globalized world and intensified competition, cannot overlook the potential risks associated with ignoring and opportunities associated with embracing the technological innovations in the era of fourth industrial revolution (Kant, 2020).

Davidson et al. (2016) argue in favor of disruptive potentialities of blockchain in a centralized system coordinating information. Umeh (2016) argues that corporations, irrespective of their sectors, have shown interest in blockchain in awe of its huge potentials which can drive their digital transformation and provide solutions to their real-life problems. Here, studies suggest that there is a need to evaluate its suitability against the use cases requirements before adopting such solutions enabled by blockchain (Lo et al., 2017). Nonetheless, Casino et al. (2019) caution against the limitedness of the frameworks in terms of their numbers developed in the scientific literature to evaluate the suitability of such applications enabled by blockchain. Healthcare system can derive value from the blockchain for: privacy of the sensitive medical information; ability to reduce redundancies by bringing insurance companies, hospital billing departments, patients, and lenders on a single blockchain; innovations in preventative care and community-based models related to healthcare enabling a synergy; and risk mitigation using smart contracts in the sharing of sensitive data sharing and avoiding compliance breaches (IET Healthcare, 2019). It is notable that the level of understating and the hype around blockchain have attracted huge attention to use it wrongfully to solve any problem, rendering it to fail considerably against the exaggerated expectations (Iansiti & Lakhani, 2017). These failures caution not to take the hype lightly at a time of its fast expansion and higher usage in comparison to others in recent times. Yet, this must not be forgotten that it has affected human life increasingly but not highly aggressively, as posits Brenner (2007). Casino et al. (2019), however, point out the attention of corporations in making more investment in blockchain perceiving its potentialities in decentralizing their architectures and reducing transaction costs foreseeing its inherent higher safety, transparency, and fastness, considering it no longer as a hype. At a time when governments are yet to formulate suitable monitoring mechanism for blockchain ecosystem to protect the stakeholders' interest, it is also notable that there are several concerns, e.g., necessity of "Proof of Work" consensus, which cause wastage of energy and slow performance (Vukolić, 2016) resulting into extra expenditure for healthcare system. Further, Casino et al. (2019) outline the main limitation of the blockchain which is the waste of mining network resources giving rise to the concerns related to the ways of minimizing energy consumption and applying the computational power to useful processing of data. However, they highlight that majority of blockchains including but not limited to Ethereum have started to shift to proof-of-stake (PoS) protocol as it significantly reduces power consumption while improving scalability.

However, Casino et al. (2019), pointing at the increasing interest of academics in blockchain-enabled applications identifying their sectoral classification, their suitability for creating value without ignoring various limitations, and providing a future research roadmap vis-à-vis avenues – challenges – opportunities as the three main research streams seeking their attention for further research in future, caution that any review cannot be exhaustive due to novelty and constant fast-paced growth. They also warn that despite the wider deployment of blockchain applications, addressing multiple issues and concerns is essentially required in order to make it more scalable, efficient, and more durable. Casino et al. (2019) posit that the individual features offered by blockchain-enabled applications might not be unique keeping in view that their different mechanisms are popularly known but their combinations

RESORCE	ATTAINING COMPETITIVE ADVANTAGE				SUSTAINING COMPETITIVE ADVANTAGE				LIEKLIHOOD
	Cost Leadership	Differentiation	Focus (Cost)	Focus (Differentiation)	V (Valuable)	R (Rare)	I (Inimitable)	N (Non-substitutable)	Attributes ← / Outcome ↓
	No	No	No	No	No	No	No	No	Competitive Disadvantage
	Yes*				Yes	No	No	No	Competitive Parity
					Yes	Yes	No	No	Transient Competitive Advantage
	*Any one or the combination of more than one				Yes	Yes	Yes	No	Transient Competitive Advantage
					Yes	Yes	Yes	Yes	Sustained Competitive Advantage
Blockchain in Healthcare System	Yes*				Yes	Yes	Yes	Yes	Sustained Competitive Advantage

FIGURE 1.2 Strategic potentialities of blockchain in the healthcare system. (Adapted from Barney (1991) and Porter (1980).)

make them idiosyncratic fuelling the greater interest by a plethora of industries. With more maturity in days to come, they can become useful for greater number of industries and domains to facilitate selection of the suitable blockchain and corresponding mechanisms customizing them according to their actual needs. Blockchain can be used by healthcare organizations in finding solutions to any problem following "problem first-technology second" approach which is considered to fetch competitiveness, maintain Vitso et al. (2017), considering that the selection process of appropriate technology is believed to be an important factor for competitive advantage.

Figure 1.2 illustrates the strategic potentialities of blockchain in the healthcare system based on the discussion in this chapter.

1.6 LIMITATIONS OF THE CHAPTER

Keeping in view of the broadness of the scope of this chapter, the intention was never to make an investigation into the technical aspects of blockchain. The chapter therefore does not develop and present the technicalities involved. The objective of the chapter was also not to cover its programming aspects or developing any product for the healthcare system using blockchain. The chapter covers only the strategic aspects with very little technical and other details which were relevant to create the background for easy comprehensibility for any reader with little technical knowledge. Moreover, the chapter attempted to discuss blockchain with a reference to the context of healthcare system without touching upon all aspects of healthcare system.

1.7 CONCLUSION

The healthcare system needs to handle tremendous competing pressure by developing ability to utilize the continuously growing health data optimally for getting new insights and driving transformation to a more patient-centric healthcare system. With each passing day, the pressure on organizations in any sector to remain ahead in the battle of competitiveness is getting more intense and organizations in healthcare system are no exceptions. They are under continuous compulsion to customize their products, services, and processes aligned with the growing stakeholders' expectations. Effective use of blockchain, an emerging technological innovation, offers huge potentialities as an intangible strategic resource through the transfer of controlling authority of the patients themselves of their personal sensitive medical data stored therein, also opening up opportunities for organizations to acquire cost leadership and/or differentiation. The strategic attributes of this intangible resource with its idiosyncrasies can help organizations in healthcare system attain sustained competitive advantage with more cost-efficiency and greater differentiation than rivals not using it which can be a visible distinction. While blockchain has the potential to manage accessibility to electronic medical records stored on the cloud, it can improve interoperability without any compromise of data security and privacy and can ensure compliance with regulations more efficiently.

Future research needs to focus on the strategic aspects of blockchain in healthcare system, comprising a complex system of interconnected entities in majority of the countries, as to how it can fill the chasm between needs, priorities, practices, and models by sensing the threats and opportunities, seizing the opportunities and reconfiguring resources and capabilities, and making a suitable decision in anticipation of the future trends. Healthcare system has witnessed a rapid increase in the cost of its delivery with highest contributions of administrative costs. Here, blockchain offers strategic potentialities as the next big disruptive technological innovation in healthcare system especially with respect to interoperability and portability of patients' data, delivery of affordable but quality services and administration addressing major concerns of the industry, provided the acceptance of blockchain within the healthcare ecosystem happens smoothly. The experience with blockchain-enabled applications makes one believe that with the idiosyncrasies in terms of higher security and accessibility, blockchain can be immensely useful in the healthcare system in different areas including but not limited to storage, and sharing of medical and insurance-related information not only at static hospitals but also in virtual presence of healthcare entities and clinical trials. Though there is inadequacy of relevant research with respect to strategic use of blockchain in the healthcare system currently, the few research along with their significantly useful findings are hinting at the possibility of a situation when patients would be having complete authority over their own medical records transforming the system as a patient-centric system reversing the hierarchical structure. Its idiosyncratic features make it a potentially valuable technology for healthcare system which can help it in living up to the continuously rising expectations of varied regularly interacting stakeholders. Blockchain in its infancy in healthcare system needs to be funded through incentives for ensuring open-mindedness among stakeholders toward experimentation in real-world environment to reap the rich harvest of its potential benefits. While the awareness needs to be raised in the healthcare system, better skills and expertise also need to be built not only by providing adequate research funding but nurturing start-ups properly. Entities in healthcare system need to make efforts to use it for process optimization and experience gaining through small-scale use cases to be used later on a larger scale for higher benefits. Future research needs to supplement these efforts which would offer much-needed support to the issues and concerns of interoperability, scalability, data security, and data privacy in healthcare system.

REFERENCES

Barney, J. B. (1991). Firm resources and sustained competitive advantage. *Journal of Management, 17*(1), 99–120.

Barney, J. B. (2001). Resource-based theories of competitive advantage: A ten-year retrospective on the resource-based view. *Journal of Management, 27*(6), 643–650.

Bdiwi, R., De Runz, C., Faiz, S., & Cherif, A. A. (2017). Towards a new ubiquitous learning environment based on blockchain technology. *Proceedings – IEEE 17th International Conference on Advanced Learning Technologies, ICALT 2017*, Timisoara, Romania, pp. 101–102.

Benchoufi, M., & Ravaud, P. (2017). Blockchain technology for improving clinical research quality. *Trials, 18*(1), 335. doi: 10.1186/s13063-017-2035-z.

Bharadwaj, A. (2000). A resource-based perspective on information technology capability and firm performance: An empirical investigation. *Management Information Systems Quarterly, 24*(1), 169–196.

Boucher, P. (2016). What if blockchain technology revolutionised voting? Scientific Foresight Unit (STOA), European Parliamentary Research Service.

Brenner, S. W. (2007). *Law in an Era of 'Smart' Technology.* Oxford University Press, Oxford.

Casino, F., Dasaklis, T. K., & Patsakis, C. (2019). A systematic literature review of blockchain-based applications: Current status, classification and open issues. *Telematics and Informatics, 36*, 55–81. doi: 10.1016/j.tele.2018.11.006.

Chen, G., Xu, B., Lu, M., & Chen, N.-S. (2018). Exploring blockchain technology and its potential applications for education. *Smart Learning Environments, 5*(1), 1. doi: 10.1186/s40561-017-0050-x.

Chen, H. S., Jarrell, J. T., Carpenter, K. A., Cohen, D. S., & Huang, X. (2019). Blockchain in healthcare: A patient-centered model. *Biomedical Journal of Scientific & Technical Research, 20*(3), 15017–15022.

Christidis, K., & Devetsikiotis, M. (2016). Blockchains and smart contracts for the internet of things. *IEEE Access, 4*, 2292–2303.

COCIR. (2017). Beyond the hype of blockchain in healthcare (Issue December). https://www.cocir.org/media-centre/publications/article/beyond-the-hype-of-blockchain-in-healthcare.html.

Davidson, S., De Filippi, P., & Potts, J. (2016). Economics of blockchain. *SSRN Electronic Journal.* doi: 10.2139/ssrn.2744751.

Deloitte. (2016). Blockchain applications in insurance. Turning a buzzword into a breakthrough for health and life insurers. https://www2.deloitte.com/us/en/pages/life-sciences-and-health-care/articles/blockchain-in-insurance.html.

Falle, S., Rauter, R., Engert, S., & Baumgartner, R. J. (2016). Sustainability management with the sustainability balanced scorecard in SMEs: Findings from an Austrian case study. *Sustainability, 8*(6), 545.

Grech, A., & Camilleri, A. F. (2017). Blockchain in education. JRC Working Papers JRC108255; Joint Research Centre.

Grey Healthcare. (2017). Blockchain: What's next for healthcare?

Hitt, M. A., Ireland, R. D., Camp, S. M., & Sexton, D. L. (2001). Strategic entrepreneurship: Entrepreneurial strategies for wealth creation. *Strategic Management Journal, 22*(6), 479–492.

Hou, H. (2017). The application of blockchain technology in E-government in China. *26th International Conference on Computer Communications and Networks, ICCCN 2017*, Vancouver, Canada.

Hoy, M. B. (2017). An introduction to the blockchain and its implications for libraries and medicine. *Medical Reference Services Quarterly, 36*(3), 273–279.

Iansiti, M., & Lakhani, K. R. (2017). The truth about blockchain. Harvard Business Review. https://hbr.org/2017/01/the-truth-about-blockchain.

IBM Corp. (2016). Making blockchain real for business. Explained with high security business network service.

Idrees, S. M., Nowostawski, M., & Jameel, R. (2021). Blockchain-based digital contact tracing apps for COVID-19 pandemic management: Issues, challenges, solutions, and future directions. *JMIR Medical Informatics*, 9(2), e25245.

IET Healthcare. (2019). Blockchain in healthcare.

Ind AS. (2015). Indian Accounting Standard (Ind AS) 38 Intangible Assets. Ministry of Corporate Affairs, Govt. of India. http://mca.gov.in/Ministry/pdf/INDAS38.pdf.

Kant, N. (2020). Blockchain: A resource of competitive advantage in open and distance learning system. In R. C. Sharma, H. Yildirim, & G. Kurubacak (Eds.), *Blockchain Technology Applications in Education* (pp. 127–152). IGI Global, Pennsylvania. doi: 10.4018/978-1-5225-9478-9.ch007.

Kant, N., & Anjali, K. (2020). Climate Strategy Proactivity (CSP): A stakeholders-centric concept. In W. L. Filho, A. M. Azul, L. Brandli, A. L. Salvia, & T. Wall (Eds.), *Partnerships for the Goals, Encyclopedia of the UN Sustainable Development Goals (Living Reference)* (pp. 1–16). Springer Nature, Basingstoke. doi: 10.1007/978-3-319-71067-9_121-1.

Khezr, S., Yassine, A., & Benlamri, R. (2019). Blockchain technology in healthcare: A comprehensive review and directions for future research. *Applied Science*, 9(1736), 1–28. doi: 10.3390/app9091736.

Klewitz, J., & Hansen, E. G. (2014). Sustainability-oriented innovation of SMEs: A systematic review. *Journal of Cleaner Production*, 65, 57–75.

Lo, S. K., Xu, X., Chiam, Y. K., & Lu, Q. (2017). Evaluating suitability of applying blockchain. *Proceedings of the IEEE International Conference on Engineering of Complex Computer Systems, ICECCS*, Fukuoka, pp. 158–161. doi: 10.1109/ICECCS.2017.26

Nakamoto, S. (2008). *Bitcoin: A Peer-to-Peer Electronic Cash System.* https://bitcoin.org/bitcoin.pdf.

Nguyen, Q. K. (2016). Blockchain: A financial technology for future sustainable development. *Proceedings – 3rd International Conference on Green Technology and Sustainable Development, GTSD 2016*, Kaohsiung, Taiwan, pp. 51–54.

Noizat, P. (2015). Blockchain electronic vote. In D. L. K. Chuen (Ed.), *Handbook of Digital Currency: Bitcoin, Innovation, Financial Instruments, and Big Data* (pp. 453–461), Elsevier, Amsterdam.

Nugent, T., Upton, D., & Cimpoesu, M. (2016). Improving data transparency in clinical trials using blockchain smart contracts, *F1000Research 5*.

Peteraf, M. A. (1993). The cornerstones of competitive advantage: A resource-based view. *Strategic Management Journal*, 14, 179–191.

Porter, M. E. (1980). *Competitive Strategy.* Free Press, New York.

Porter, M. E. (1985). *The Competitive Advantage: Creating and Sustaining Superior Performance.* Free Press, New York.

Porter, M. E. (1990). *The Competitive Advantage of Nations,* (Republished with a new introduction, 1998). Free Press, New York.

Potenza, A. (2017). Can renewable power offset bitcoin's massive energy demands?

Puthal, D., Malik, N., Mohanty, S. P., Kougianos, E., & Yang, C. (2018). The blockchain as a decentralized security framework [future directions]. *IEEE Consumer Electronices Magazine*, 7(2), 18–21.

Reed, M. (2005). Reflections on the "realist turn" in organization and management studies. *Journal of Management Studies*, 42(8), 1621–1644.

Swan, M. (2015). *Blockchain: Blueprint for a New Economy* (1st ed.). O'Reilly Media, Sebastopol, CA.

Teece, D. J. (2007). Explicating dynamic capabilities: The nature and microfoundations of (sustainable) enterprise performance. *Strategic Management Journal, 28*(13), 1319–1350.

Teece, D., & Pisano, G. (1994). The dynamic capabilities of firms: An Introduction. *Industrial and Corporate Change, 3*(3), 537–556.

Teece, D. J., Pisano, G., & Shuen, A. (1997). Dynamic capabilities and strategic management. *Strategic Management Journal, 18*(7), 509–533.

Umeh, J. (2016). Blockchain double bubble or double trouble? *ITNOW, 58*(1), 58–61.

Underwood, S. (2016). Blockchain beyond bitcoin. *Communications of the ACM, 59*(11), 15–17.

Vitso, M., Joar, B., Harkestad, G., & Krogh, S. (2017). A study on blockchain technology as a resource for competitive advantage (dissertation). Norwegian University of Science and Technology.

Vukolić, M. (2016). The quest for scalable blockchain fabric: Proof-of-work vs. BFT replication. *Lecture Notes in Computer Science (Including Subseries Lecture Notes in Artificial Intelligence and Lecture Notes in Bioinformatics), 9591*, 112–125. doi: 10.1007/978-3-319-39028-4_9.

Weerawardena, J., & Mavondo, F. T. (2011). Capabilities, innovation and competitive advantage. *Industrial Marketing Management, 40*(8), 1220–1223.

White, G. R. T. (2017). Future applications of blockchain in business and management: A delphi study. *Strategic Change, 26*(5), 439–451.

Xu, Y., Zhao, S., Kong, L., Zheng, Y., Zhang, S., & Li, Q. (2017). ECBC: A high performance educational certificate blockchain with efficient query. In *Lecture Notes in Computer Science (Including Subseries Lecture Notes in Artificial Intelligence and Lecture Notes in Bioinformatics)*, vol. 10580 LNCS (pp. 288–304).

Yaeger, K., Martini, M., Rasouli, J., & Costa, A. (2019). Emerging blockchain technology solutions for modern healthcare infrastructure. *Journal of Scientific Innovation in Medicine, 2*(1). doi:10.29024/jsim.7.

Zhao, J. L., Fan, S., & Yan, J. (2016). Overview of business innovations and research opportunities in blockchain and introduction to the special issue. *Financial Innovation, 2*(1), 28.

Zhu, H., & Zhou, Z. Z. (2016). Analysis and outlook of applications of blockchain technology to equity crowdfunding in China. *Financial Innovation, 2*(1), 1–29.

2 Blockchain Technology and Its Applications in the Healthcare Sector

Ishfaq Hussain Rather
Jawaharlal Nehru University

Sheikh Mohammad Idrees
Norwegian University of Science and Technology

CONTENTS

2.1 INTRODUCTION

Blockchain is the new technological revolution that will impact almost every human being in society. It is the technology behind the famous Bitcoin [1] and other cryptocurrencies which have proved that Blockchain has a potential that could reshape all aspects of our society and its operations. The features of Blockchain are numerous such as the public distributed ledger which records transactions and provides decentralized transactional data management. It operates on a peer-to-peer network

DOI: 10.1201/9781003141471-2

without any central monitoring authority. A transaction recorded in the ledger can never be changed. Identities of users are kept hidden and private. This system is secure as there is no central failure point that may disrupt the functioning of the entire network. It provides increased capacity having thousands of computers working together that can produce more power than a few centralized nodes.

The famous white paper [1] by "Satoshi Nakamoto" published in October 2008 proposed concept of the Bitcoin and in the next year there was an open-source implementation of Bitcoin which gave rise to three different generations of Blockchain technologies: (a) Blockchain 1.0, (b) Blockchain 2.0, and (c) Blockchain 3.0. Bitcoins or the other Blockchain-based cryptocurrencies represent Blockchain 1.0, which is the first generation of Blockchain. Smart properties and smart contracts like Ethereum [2], QTUM, and NEO [3] refer to Blockchain 2.0 generation. Blockchain 3.0 constitutes the applications of Blockchain in non-financial organizations. Efforts are being made to use this technology in industries other than finance. Healthcare is considered as one such area where Blockchain can have significant impacts.

2.2 BLOCKCHAIN ARCHITECTURE

The architecture of Blockchain reveals the connection between nodes in the network which are involved in transaction and validation purposes. There are three types of Blockchain architectures [4]: (a) Permissioned Blockchain, (b) Unpermissioned Blockchain, and (c) Consortium or federated Blockchain. In permissioned Blockchain, the network already knows the nodes involved in the Blockchain, e.g., Hyperledger Fabric and Ripple, which are also private Blockchains. Management of data access authorization by the network is strict in them. The verification of every transaction in the network is done by the companies or organizations only. Other type of Blockchain known as unpermissioned ledger is the blockchain in which the network is open to any individual or organizational node. Here, the transaction can be validated by any member of the network and any member can participate in its process of approval through the consensus algorithm, e.g., Bitcoin or Ethereum. Consortium or federated Blockchain is the third type of Blockchain network suited for those organizations where there is a need for both private and public Blockchains. In this Blockchain, multiple organizations maintain the central authority, and they are involved in providing access to pre-selected nodes for reading, writing, and auditing the Blockchain. The decentralized authority is maintained as there is no single authority governing the control.

Figure 2.1 shows the Blockchain architecture. It consists of a collection of blocks, which contain transaction information. Every block has a parent block except the first block which is called the genesis block. The block hash value is contained in the header of the next block, and the hash value of that block is contained in the header of the block next and so on making it a chain of blocks [5]. A header of the block contains the following information:

(i) **Block Version**: Block version refers to the collection of validation rules.
(i) **Merkel Tree Root (MTR) Hash**: MTR is the hash value of all the transactions that are part of a block
(ii) **Time Stamp**: Time stamp indicates the current time in seconds

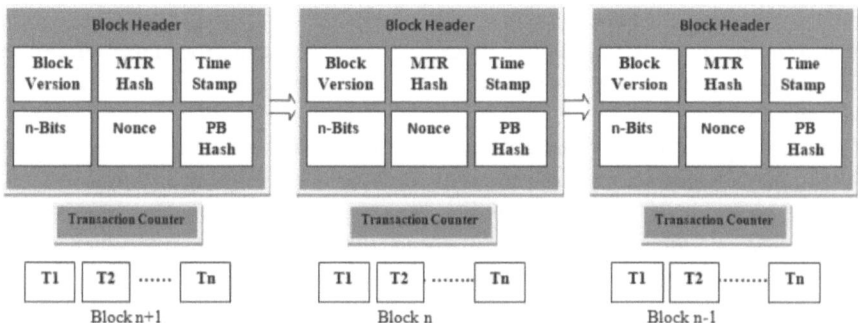

FIGURE 2.1   Shows the Blockchain architecture.

(iii) **n-Bits**: It is the target threshold of a valid block hash
(iv) **Nonce**: This is a 4-bit field, which increases when every hash value is calculated. It starts from 0.
(v) **Parent Block Hash**: Parent block Hash contains the previous block hash
value.

Transactions and transaction counter together make the body of block. The number
of transactions in a block depends on the block size and the size of each transaction.
To maintain the authenticity of transactions, "asymmetric cryptography mechanism"
[6] is used. For trustworthy communication between the nodes, digital signatures
based on asymmetric cryptography are used.

2.3   BLOCKCHAIN IN HEALTHCARE

Blockchain is growing rapidly in different organizations and industries. Healthcare is
one such industry in which significant numbers of applications have been identified
where Blockchain can bring revolution.

In healthcare industry, huge data is generated, accessed, and stored daily. It is
critical for the healthcare industry to access, edit, and trust the data generated from
different activities in the healthcare organization. Certain properties like interoperability, information sharing, data integrity, provenance, and access control must be
followed for patients' privacy and data exchange. These properties are necessary for
building trust in the healthcare ecosystem. Access control can be defined as the trust
between the data owner and the entities who store it. These entities are the servers
given the responsibility to enforce access control policies.

Interoperability is the potential to share and exchange information very easily
among different stakeholders. The aim is to optimize the health of individuals and
populations. Data provenance is the record of historical sequence of events. It prevents data manipulation by providing auditibility and transparency of all data that is
collected, processed, and accessed by the researchers. Data integrity can be defined
as the degree to which the integrity or the quality of data is met.

There is a huge demand for real-world data from different organizations and
research institutions. Any unauthorized data sharing and stealing of sensitive data

gradually destroys the trust of public in the healthcare. Also, illegal practices within the healthcare ecosystem (like fake drugs, lack of skills, and procedures) erode the same trust. There is a need to consider an alternate approach to overcome the problems mentioned above.

Blockchain could be an alternate approach because of its attributes like decentralization, distribution, and data integrity. It could also be utilized to improve and obtain a higher level of interoperability, access control, provenance, information sharing, and data integrity [7] among different stakeholders. Thus, Blockchain could be a new infrastructure that can help in building trust in healthcare industry.

2.4 APPLICATIONS OF BLOCKCHAIN IN HEALTHCARE

- **Data Sharing Among Different Stakeholders**
- **Data Management**
- **Health Insurance Claim Settlement**
- **Patient Digital Identity**
- **Electronic Health Records (EHRs)**

2.4.1 DATA SHARING AMONG DIFFERENT STAKEHOLDERS

Sharing of healthcare data among the stakeholders like hospitals, clinical institutes, insurance companies, and organizations which do research and development can improve the quality of healthcare providers. There are different challenges that need to be taken care of before the data is shared. The first challenge is data security, as more and more data is stored in the public cloud where there are risks of data exposure. The second challenge is that patients may not have access to their health records always. Thus, sharing their own data with unknown parties is impossible for them. The third challenge is the centralized architecture of current systems, and thus the central authority needs to be trustworthy.

Blockchain technology can play a crucial role in providing user-centric access control, security, and privacy [8] in data sharing infrastructure. Some contributions of Blockchain for data sharing are mentioned below.

MedBlock, a Blockchain-based data management system, is proposed in [9] for handling patient information. Electronic medical records (EMRs) are efficiently accessed and retrieved through the distributed ledger of MedBlock. Thus the problem of data being scattered among different databases is avoided. Hospitals may get to know about the medical history of a patient in advance through Blockchain-based data sharing and collaboration. In addition, MedBlocks provide high information security and sharing.

In Ref. [10], the authors have presented a new approach based on logging system on OpenNCP for the exchange of ehealth data across the border. They have been able to provide security of data, traceability and liability support within OpenNCP infrastructure. In Paper [11], the authors have presented a Blockchain-based application called "Healthcare Data Gateway (HGD) for patients to own, control and share their own data easily and securely without violating the privacy". It is a patient-centric model because they own and control their data. A record management system based on Blockchain for handling SMRs is discussed in Ref. [12]. The system is called MedRec. It provides easy access to patient's medical records across different healthcare providers. With the help of unique Blockchain properties, MedRec provides safe and secure management of sensitive information sharing.

2.4.2   DATA MANAGEMENT

Data generated in Healthcare industry is growing rapidly. It is the core concern of different institutions to prevent security and privacy of data from malicious users because this has resulted in loss of reputation and capital of many institutions. Blockchain technology can help in providing data access to different healthcare data users on the basis of privileges allocated to them. Paper [13] proposes a "controllable Blockchain data management (CBDM) model that can be deployed in cloud environment". The model helps to address the lack of control on the posted ledgers. A special node introduced by this model called Authority Node (AN) allows the users to prevent any malicious actions even in a majority attack. Philippe Genestier et al. [14] introduce patient consent management using intrinsic features like decentralization, built-in consensus, and cryptographic of Blockchain technology. The consent management function is redefined by adding a new feature that provides finer grain to patients to manage their own consents. At the time of emergency, the patient is unable to provide access of personal health records (PHR) to the staff. Blockchain-based frameworks are also used for providing temper protection applications by considering the policies that involve identifying extensible access control, auditing, and temper resistance in an emergency scenario.

2.4.3   HEALTH INSURANCE CLAIM SETTLEMENT

Health insurance is provided to ensure care and protect the assets of an individual from loss due to accidents, medical emergency, or for the treatment of any disease. It may cover the doctor visits, medical expenses, and surgical expenses based on the type of insurance cover acquired. The insurance claim is submitted to the companies. They begin a thorough review as soon as they receive a claim. Sometimes, a small mistake such as misspelled name of the patient may reject a claim. Currently, many claims get rejected due to small mistakes as mentioned in Ref. [15], 22% claims get rejected because the insurer never received them, and sometimes the information provided is incomplete and the proof to claim is inadequate.

Blockchain technology-based smart contracts are helpful for automating the settlement process by making claims transparent to the provider and insurer. It thus exposes the potential error and frauds. One more benefit of these smart contracts is that they ensure the involved participants are notified properly as policies or rules change.

2.4.4   PATIENT DIGITAL IDENTITY

Patient identification matching is the fundamental component in health information exchange, which helps uniquely in retrieving patient information in healthcare database. It is very hard to match patient data accurately despite the increased development effort. Patient identity mismatch can lead to incorrect medical data.

An identity management system that can unify patient identification schemes used by different care providers is needed to overcome patient matching problems. Blockchain technology incorporates decentralized and unified identity system. Patient identities can be represented by cryptographically secured addresses. The addresses are linked to a key that is unique, and it can verify the ownership of an address without revealing any personal information about the individual [16].

2.4.5   ELECTRONIC HEALTH RECORDS (EHRs)

Electronic health record (EHRs) is a patient data storage method for storing data like clinical notes and laboratory results by healthcare providers. The issues in paper-based records were eliminated by EHR systems. It enhanced the patient safety by preventing errors and providing easy and increased information access. EHR systems are working in number of hospitals around the world, mainly to provide functions like medical data storage, managing appointment of patients, billing and accounts, lab tests. The goal of the EHR system is to provide secure and sharable patient data across different platforms. Despite being the popular method of patient data storage among healthcare organizations, the system faces certain problems like interoperability, information asymmetry, and data breaches [17].

Blockchain-based personal health records (PHRs) are patient-centric applications used for managing patient's data that are the actual data owners, to access and manage it. Blockchain-based PHRs help patients to monitor how the data related to their health is shared and used, verify how accurate their health information is, and also help to correct any misinformation in their record.

2.5   CHALLENGES AND LIMITATIONS OF BLOCKCHAIN BASED TECHNOLOGIES

Blockchain is an emerging technology that has applications in various sectors of human society. However, there are some challenges with this technology that need to be addressed. Some of the major challenges are (a) data security and privacy, (b) interoperability, (c) system evolvability, (d) scalability, and (f) data storage.

- **Data Security and Privacy**

- **Interoperability**

- **System Evolvability**

- **Scalability**

- **Data Storage**

2.5.1 DATA SECURITY AND PRIVACY

Public Blockchains are secure because of the authenticity and traceability of all the transactions. Despite the data being cryptographically secured, there are chances that linking together enough data could reveal the identification of the owner and the data related to him [18]. The risks of security breaches are also possible from international malicious attackers and government bodies that may compromise with patient's privacy.

2.5.2 INTEROPERABILITY

No standard exists for Blockchain-based applications developed on different platforms to interoperate in healthcare industry. Moving healthcare sector toward the Blockchain technology will require system to collaborate between medical and scientific communities.

2.5.3 SYSTEM EVOLVABILITY

Blockchain technology has a feature that is immutable, which means that the data once saved to the Blockchain cannot be erased or modified. Thus, the applications that are based on Blockchain technology with storage decentralized, modification of data is difficult. This may prove counterproductive when the patient medical history needs to be erased. Thus, Blockchain technology needs to support system evolution in healthcare applications.

2.5.4 SCALABILITY

Scalability is a major challenge in Blockchain-based healthcare applications with respect to the volume of data involved. It may lead to serious performance degradation as the volume of data increases. Thus, as more and more patients are added, the performance and speed of the Blockchain applications will become exponentially difficult to run.

2.5.5 DATA STORAGE

In healthcare applications, an enormous amount of data is generated on daily basis. These applications serve a huge number of participants such as healthcare providers, patients, billing agents, and so on. With increase in date volume, there is an enormous overhead incurred particularly when data is not normalized carefully. Storage becomes costly as the data increases which may ultimately lead access operations to fail. For Example, the "Gas Limit" in Ethereum public Blockchain defines the capacity limits of data operations to prevent attacks manifest through infinite looping. Thus in order to minimize the data storage requirement, without compromising on personal health records of the patients, is one of the main goals for future design consideration.

2.6 FUTURE RESEARCH DIRECTIONS

Healthcare industry is a complex domain; applying Blockchain technology-based systems can be robust and effective. Healthcare systems face interoperability challenges. The interoperable architecture that can be created in Blockchain would be helpful throughout many healthcare applications which face data sharing and communication challenges. It is an open research problem to design an interoperable ecosystem without compromising security and data confidentiality in healthcare systems.

Further research engagements are needed to improve data security, scalability, and speed of healthcare applications based on Blockchain. This will increase the confidence and trust of the stakeholders in this technology. To apply Blockchain technology in the healthcare industry, research on efficient software practices to educate as well as train the engineers about the potential of blockchain technology and its limitations is also needed.

2.7 CONCLUSION

Nowadays, Blockchain is gaining a lot of attention from different individuals and organizations because of its capability of transforming traditional industry with its multiple features mentioned in Ref. [19]. Blockchain technology is expected to revolutionize the healthcare industry by reshaping its operations. In this chapter, various Blockchain applications in the healthcare industry have been discussed. This research chapter has presented the current research in this area and discussed how Blockchain will empower the patient by making him the owner of his data. In addition, the challenges and limitations of Blockchain applications in healthcare are also discussed. Therefore, this chapter concludes by discussing some future directions and open research problems in the healthcare industry due to Blockchain applications.

REFERENCES

1. Nakamoto, S. (2008). Bitcoin: A peer-to-peer electronic cash system. Retrieved from https://bitcoin.org/bitcoin.pdf.
2. Vujičić, D., Jagodić, D., & Ranđić, S. (2018, March). Blockchain technology, bitcoin, and ethereum: A brief overview. *In 2018 17th International Symposium Infoteh-Jahorina (Infoteh)*, (pp. 1–6). IEEE.

3. Agbo, C. C., Mahmoud, Q. H., & Eklund, J. M. (2019, June). Blockchain technology in healthcare: A systematic review. In *Healthcare* (Vol. 7, No. 2, p. 56). Multidisciplinary Digital Publishing Institute, Basel.

4. Hussien, H. M., Yasin, S. M., Udzir, S. N. I., Zaidan, A. A., & Zaidan, B. B. (2019). A systematic review for enabling of develop a Blockchain technology in healthcare application: Taxonomy, substantially analysis, motivations, challenges, recommendations and future direction. *Journal of Medical Systems, 43*(10), 1–35.

5. Feng, Q., He, D., Zeadally, S., Khan, M. K., & Kumar, N. (2019). A survey on privacy protection in blockchain system. *Journal of Network and Computer Applications, 126*, 45–58.

6. Aung, Y. N., & Tantidham, T. (2017, November). Review of ethereum: Smart home case study. *In 2017 2nd International Conference on Information Technology (INCIT)* (pp. 1–4). IEEE.

7. Idrees, S. M., Nowostawski, M., & Jameel, R. (2021). Blockchain-based digital contact tracing apps for COVID-19 pandemic management: Issues, challenges, solutions, and future directions. *JMIR Medical Informatics, 9*(2), e25245.

8. Idrees, S. M., Nowostawski, M., Jameel, R., & Mourya, A. K. (2021). Privacy-preserving. In: P. Churi, A. Pawar, & A. A. Elngar (Eds.), *Data Protection and Privacy in Healthcare: Research and Innovations* (p. 109). CRC Press, Boca Raton, FL.

9. Fan, K., Wang, S., Ren, Y., Li, H., & Yang, Y. (2018). Medblock: Efficient and secure medical data sharing via blockchain. *Journal of Medical Systems, 42*(8), 1–11.

10. Staffa, M., Sgaglione, L., Mazzeo, G., Coppolino, L., D'Antonio, S., Romano, L., ... & Komnios, I. (2018). An OpenNCP-based solution for secure eHealth data exchange. *Journal of Network and Computer Applications, 116*, 65–85.

11. Yue, X., Wang, H., Jin, D., Li, M., & Jiang, W. (2016). Healthcare data gateways: found healthcare intelligence on blockchain with novel privacy risk control. *Journal of Medical Systems, 40*(10), 1–8.

12. Azaria, A., Ekblaw, A., Vieira, T., & Lippman, A. (2016, August). Medrec: Using blockchain for medical data access and permission management. In *2016 2nd International Conference on Open and Big Data (OBD)* (pp. 25–30). IEEE.

13. Zhu, L., Wu, Y., Gai, K., & Choo, K. K. R. (2019). Controllable and trustworthy Blockchain-based cloud data management. *Future Generation Computer Systems, 91*, 527–535.

14. Genestier, P., Zouarhi, S., Limeux, P., Excoffier, D., Prola, A., Sandon, S., & Temerson, J. M. (2017). Blockchain for consent management in the eHealth environment: A nugget for privacy and security challenges. *Journal of the International Society for Telemedicine and eHealth, 5*, GKR-e24.

15. 5 Key challenges in medical billing industry, Retrieved March 01, 2018, from https://www.invensis.net/blog/5-key-challenges-in-medical-billing-industry/.

16. Zhang, P., Schmidt, D. C., White, J., & Lenz, G. (2018). Blockchain technology use cases in healthcare. In *Advances in Computers* (Vol. 111, pp. 1–41). Elsevier, Amsterdam.

17. Shahnaz, A., Qamar, U., & Khalid, A. (2019). Using Blockchain for electronic health records. *IEEE Access, 7*, 147782–147795.

18. Radanović, I., & Likić, R. (2018). Opportunities for use of Blockchain technology in medicine. *Applied Health Economics and Health Policy, 16*(5), 583–590.

19. hezr, S., Moniruzzaman, M., Yassine, A., & Benlamri, R. (2019). Blockchain technology in healthcare: A comprehensive review and directions for future research. *Applied Sciences, 9*(9), 1736.

3 An Overview of Blockchain Technology Concepts from a Modern Perspective

Ana Carolina Borges Monteiro, Reinaldo Padilha França, Yuzo Iano, and Rangel Arthur
State University of Campinas (UNICAMP)

CONTENTS

3.1 INTRODUCTION

Looking at the simple side, blockchain technology is a public ledger recording a virtual transaction, resulting in a type of record reliable, changeless, and unalterable. That is, data and information record as the number of digital currencies transacted, related to the user who sent it, the user who received it, the date when this digital transaction was fulfilled, and in which place in the ledger it is registered, relating to the financial sector (Drescher 2017, Van Rijmenam & Ryan 2018).

Blockchain stores this set of digital transactions (information) in blocks, defining each one with a time and date stamp. At each period, in general minutes or less, a new digital block respective to these transactions is created, bonding to the previous digital block. And so, the blocks form a dependent structure, i.e., blockchain. This characteristic is what consists of the blockchain appropriate for recording a virtual transaction that needs trust (Drescher 2017, Prusty 2017).

DOI: 10.1201/9781003141471-3

In blockchain technology, instead of this virtual transaction being stored on a central computer, this is arranged in different locations (thousands of computers) around the world. Since each of these on the network maintains a digital copy of the database, making it extremely safe and reliable, due there is no single point (computer or even server) of cyberattack (Crosby et al. 2016, Biswas & Muthukkumarasamy 2016).

Still it is considering that it is not possible to access the central computer (server) of the blockchain and swipe the virtual transaction records or even change it, given that each node on the blockchain network has a registration of this data. Once an attempt to alter a computer's database is identified, this node will be expelled from the blockchain network (Crosby et al. 2016, Zheng et al. 2017).

The blockchain network is made up of checking on the records of these virtual transactions on the block. Depending on the characteristics of each type of network, each computer lends its computational power to the network. Regarding the approach toward miners, who also do this check, an incentive (reward) is given to proceed to collaborate and making the blockchain network sustainable. The validation of a transaction in the digital block given by a simple majority (50% + 1) agrees that this virtual transaction is legitimate, that is, the consensus blockchain (Zheng et al. 2017, Tasatanattakool & Techapanupreeda 2018, Idrees et al. 2021).

Still it is considering that every block contains a resume of all the data inserted in it, called as hash, this content is formed by information plus a hash of the previous block plus hash of the block. Since more data is transmitted, it waits in the queue until it is possible to be inserted into a digital block. Still it is reflecting that the hash of the next block containing digital transaction data must be compatible with the hash of the previous digital block, occurring that these two digital blocks are dependent and linked on each other. In such a way, that it is not possible to make any modifications without the consent of the blockchain network as a whole (Zheng et al. 2017, Tasatanattakool & Techapanupreeda 2018).

Still it is reflecting on digital security given that the transactions carried out have a unique code, that is, a digital signature. This code is verified by the users themselves and the transaction needs to be approved in order to then be incorporated into the blockchain through a block. Surveillance and verification, consisting of an extremely important step to prevent fraud, in which all this information is made by the users logged on to the network, are the so-called miners. Still it is evaluating that another factor that contributes to the security of this process is the hashes, since each block has its own hash, i.e., a specific cryptographic signature (Tasatanattakool & Techapanupreeda 2018, Kaushik et al. 2017).

In summary, blockchain technology is distributed, public, forming a ledger that effectively records all virtual transactions in a considered "blockchain." The collective registration represents that the information is scattered and distributed among the several computers connected to the network. Still it is considering that it is a system that is possible to track the sending and receiving of information over the Internet, i.e., pieces of code generated online carrying linked information about virtual transactions (blocks) (Kaushik et al. 2017, Weber 2018).

With a view on the subject, this chapter produces an updated overview of blockchain technology, addressing its branch of application, approaching with succinct bibliographic background, summarizing the full potential of technology.

3.2 BLOCKCHAIN CONCEPT

Blockchain is a kind of database, where all information about digital transactions is stored, still considering that this large file is accessible to all users. In this way, it is possible to access this database and see a digital negotiation that took place between two people, without geolocation restrictions. However, the details about who is involved are not possible to know, since everything is encrypted, but it is known that that transaction occurred and that it is recorded (Figure 3.1) (Crosby et al. 2016, Drescher 2017).

Each block is a compound of several data related to umpteen virtual transactions having an exclusive digital signature, works as a fingerprint of the block, helping to provide more digital security to the blockchain process (hash). Hash works as a link between the digital blocks, due to each of these carrying its own hash and also of the previous digital block, creating a kind of seal, so it is possible to check and signal if any block has been changed, then invalidate it. As a result, a chain-forming link between various blocks contains information together. Each block is created at a constant rhythm and has a maximum capacity; this rhythm is similar to constancy like a beat of a song or a heart, since, in that time, several digital transactions between digital users are checked, verified, and then aggregated to the blockchain network (Drescher 2017, Zheng et al. 2017).

Still pondering that when a (legitimate) update is made, all copies are synchronized in a matter of seconds. It may even be that one or another computer disappears from the network, but it will not affect the system, since all the other nodes are still there (Prusty 2017, Weber 2018).

Hash is a mathematical function that takes a message or file and generates a code with letters and numbers, this code uses a hexadecimal basis, which represents the data sent (which can be messages or files). Essentially, it is the hash that takes a large amount of data and transforms it into a small amount of information, i.e., it is the "fingerprint"

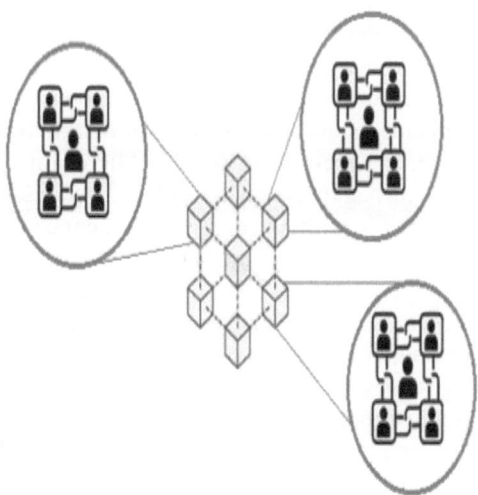

FIGURE 3.1 Connected blockchain illustration

of the file/block, still considering that when signing the content of the block, if any information is changed, the hash changes (Tasatanattakool & Techapanupreeda 2018, Applebaum et al. 2017).

Each blockchain network also has "nodes," that group participants who have the same interest; these nodes can be either transactional, which write or generate blocks, or miners, who check whether the written block is valid (Tasatanattakool & Techapanupreeda 2018, Applebaum et al. 2017).

Each of the transactions carried out has a unique code, which is verified by the users themselves and the transaction must be approved to then be incorporated into the blockchain through a block. The surveillance and verification of all this information are done by the users logged on to the network, given that this verification is an extremely important step to avoid fraud. Another factor that contributes to the digital security of this process is hashes, since each block has its own specific cryptographic signature (Drescher 2017, Gupta & Sadoghi 2019).

The greatest virtues of blockchain technology are related to network distribution and decentralization, the security of data immutability, and transparency. Still related to accessibility to any user, since everything will be registered in a large database shared with users from all over the world (Gupta & Sadoghi 2019, Zhao 2020).

3.3   BLOCKCHAIN TYPES

A public blockchain, i.e., permissionless, considers the most distributed ledgers that currently is practiced, due to any user be able to view the virtual transactions that take place and membership, consisting in a simple circumstance of downloading the required software. No one can prevent participation and anyone can get involved with the consensus mechanism (mining or staking), allowing anyone to be free to join and receive the reward for their role in obtaining consensus, given a highly decentralized network topology established around a public chain. Proof of work (PoW) causes a lot of waste, but it proved required for an open digital environment, considering the security model (Lu 2018, Gabison 2016).

Public networks at the expense of speed and performance tend to stand out in terms of resistance to censorship, consisted of great options for obtaining security guarantees in agreements and transactions, or smart contracts, for example. Regarding performance, the security-oriented public chain approach faces scalability obstacles and the throughput is relatively low. In addition, sending modifications to a blockchain network without fragmenting them can be challenging, as it is difficult for all users to agree on the proposed modifications (Lu 2018, Gabison 2016, Xu et al. 2019).

Semiprivate blockchain is related to anyone who can bond the network; however, the protocol must incorporate specific mechanisms to avoid malicious agents from obtaining an advantage anonymously (Lu 2018, Gabison 2016, Xu et al. 2019).

The blockchain is a distributed ledger technology (DLT), still reflecting that the blockchain itself is just one type of DLT, given that not all DLT is a blockchain. It is often just a computer network sharing the same database, reflecting that many times these networks are small and centralized, which is the opposite of blockchain (Gabison 2016, Xu et al. 2019, Gupta 2017).

Private blockchain establishes rules that determine who can see and write in the chain, i.e., requiring authorization. A private blockchain is not a decentralized system, considering a clear hierarchy in relation to digital control. However, it is distributed over many nodes that maintain a replica of the chain on their computational devices. This prioritizes the speed of the system, as it does not have to worry with respect to central points of possible failure, as in the public case it is ideal in circumstances where a user or company must remain in control and the data kept confidential (Gabison 2016, Xu et al. 2019, Gupta 2017).

They are more suitable for corporate use since they do not make the network accessible externally; however, the threats that PoW detains are not so harmful, considering that the identity of each participant is known and the management is done practically. In this type of context, a more efficient algorithm can be applied, selecting nodes (designated validators) to assume certain functions in the validation of transactions, involving a variety of nodes that must approve each block. Still pondering that if the nodes act maliciously, these nodes can be quickly seized and removed from the blockchain network (Xu et al. 2019, Gupta 2017, Babkin et al. 2018).

A consortium blockchain is a middle ground between private and public blockchain, combining components of both, differentiating that either system can be watched at the consensus mechanism level. Still it is relating that an open system, i.e., public blockchain, is the one where any user can validate digital blocks or a closed system (private blockchain) is the one where only a unique entity appoints digital block validators. So, a blockchain of consortia works with an equally powerful group of participants working as validators. Still it is considering that the chain's visibility can be limited just for validators, visible to the authorized user or by everyone (Xu et al. 2019, Gupta 2017, Babkin et al. 2018).

This type of blockchain would be more advantageous in a scenario in which several companies act in the same sector and need a mutual environment carrying virtual transactions or to relay data about it, as it would allow the sharing of information about their sector with other participants. So, it attenuates some of the counterparty hazard risks of a private blockchain (eliminating centralized digital control) and a small number of nodes that allow for much more effective performance than a public chain (Xu et al. 2019, Gupta 2017, Babkin et al. 2018).

3.4 CONSENSUS MECHANISM

The consensus mechanism (algorithm) is a method relating to all pairs of the blockchain network to attain a mutual agreement on the current status of the spread ledger. Achieving network reliability and establishing reliability between unknown peers in a widespread computing digital environment, ensuring that each new digital block aggregated to the blockchain is the unique description of the truth that was agreed with all nodes (Gupta 2017, Babkin et al. 2018, Cachin & Vukolić 2017).

Public (decentralized) blockchain networks are constructed as widespread systems and, since it does not depend on a central digital authority, the computers on the network must agree to validate the transactions. In this context, consensus algorithms ensure that the rules of the protocol are being fulfilled and that all virtual transactions succeed reliably (Gupta 2017, Babkin et al. 2018, Wang et al. 2018).

Using a blockchain network and algorithm as a mechanism, it is also possible to define protocol as the primary rules that will be followed. This is related to the algorithm dictate the blockchain system what steps it needs to take to agree with those rules defined by the protocol, producing the expected result. A protocol for a particular cryptocurrency determines how nodes (users) interact, how information about virtual transactions is transmitted between nodes, and what are the exigencies that the block validation is successful. Under another approach, a consensus algorithm is accountable for checking the digital fingerprint and digital signatures, acknowledging the virtual transactions, and performing the virtual validation of the digital blocks, depending on the network consensus (Gupta 2017, Babkin et al. 2018, Wang et al. 2018).

The consensus mechanism of blockchain technology comprises a couple of particular objectives, such as reaching a collaboration, agreement, cooperation, equal rights, and even validation to all nodes, and still obligatory participation of each node (user) in the digital consensus process. Thus, a consensus mechanism tends to find a mutual agreement for the entire blockchain network (Gupta 2017, Babkin et al. 2018, Wang et al. 2018).

Proof of work is employed electing a digital miner for the next-generation process of blocks, with a central idea in solving a "complex mathematical puzzle" and easily providing a decision. This specific mathematical puzzle needs a lot of computational energy and, that way, the node (user) that resolves the mathematical puzzle as quickly as possible reaches its next block. So, the more computational power the more attempts per second, the greater the chances of finding a valid solution to the mathematical problem of the next block. PoW also guarantees that miners are allowed to validate new virtual transaction blocks and aggregate them to the blockchain, if the widespread network of nodes attains consensus and gets an agreement that the solution to the mathematical problem presented is a valid proof of the effort employed in the process (Gupta 2017, Babkin et al. 2018, Gervais et al. 2016).

Proof of stake (PoS) is the most mutual option to PoW, instead of making an investment in expensive hardware to resolve a "complex puzzle," therewith digital validators invest in the system's cryptocurrencies, blocking some of their cryptocurrencies as a way of participation in the network. After that, all validators will begin to validate the blocks to bet if they find out the one that can be added to the blockchain network. PoS replaces the PoW mechanism, using the allocated capital (stake) of each participant to validate new blocks, given that the validator (forger) is decided by the investment befitting of cryptocurrency in question and not by computational power allocated to the process (Gupta 2017, Babkin et al. 2018, Li et al. 2017).

Leased proof of stake (LPoS) facilitates the maintenance of nodes through the contribution of network users, since users who do not have a node "lend" their cryptocurrencies to one so that it has more strength within the network, so that he does not necessarily need his own coins to forge. In addition, to continue with the decentralization proposal, the user can cancel the lease at any time and carry out the procedure on the same node as many times and for as long as it exists (Gupta 2017, Babkin et al. 2018, Hakak et al. 2020).

Proof of capacity requires a storage capacity from the miner; this algorithm consumes less energy and performance on the user's machines, following the same concept of PoS draw, but what gives strength to the miner is the storage capacity on the HD (Hard Disk Drive) of the machine. The more space, the more strength, and the more chance of being drawn. As any type of data can be inserted into the network, this type of algorithm can be a good proposal for streaming videos, a file library, or any other type of media platform, but with the practicality and quality of decentralization (Gupta 2017, Babkin et al. 2018, Jiang & Wu 2020).

Consensus algorithms are critical to maintaining the security and integrity of a blockchain network, providing ways for a network to reach a consensus on which version of the block is the correct one. Due to decentralization, the technology is becoming more comprehensive and bringing even more possibilities of use, because, with the proposal of immutable registration, speed in sending, receiving data, and network confirmations, the application ideas are numerous (Gupta 2017, Babkin et al. 2018, Drescher 2017, Weber 2018).

3.5   ADVANTAGES AND DISADVANTAGES

The structure in the form of blockchains makes the blockchain practically inviolable, given that in order to be able to prevent a digital invader. Availability is a great benefit, evaluating the spread structure maintains the system working even facing the possibility of one or more nodes (users) fall; in this case, missing nodes go back to the blockchain network, where these nodes are promptly updated. Regarding reliability, the data cannot be erased or changed, since the registered transactions are fulfilled and legitimate (Golosova & Romanovs 2018, Mengelkamp et al. 2018).

Regarding the aspect of transparency, virtual transactions are public, meaning that all nodes perform a check on it, still reflecting how much the encryption procedures imply that the users of the system do not demand to be detected. However, there is still the possibility of link virtual identities, if this aspect ensures that only authentic users take part in the virtual transaction (Mengelkamp et al. 2018, Kim et al. 2018).

When carrying out a transaction on the blockchain, it is possible to trust that the transactions will be fulfilled as determined by the protocol (rules), still considering the integrity, eliminating the requirement for intermediaries, and making the whole process more reliable (Mengelkamp et al. 2018, Gabison 2016).

Regarding data quality, due the data is complete, it is dated, it has consistency, it is absolutely accurate and available to everyone. Still pondering that because they are encrypted, decentralized, and public, the information contained in the blockchain becomes more resistant to attacks by third parties; this generates more durability and longevity, resulting in more lasting information (Drescher 2017, Weber 2018, Jiang & Wu 2020, Idrees et al. 2021a).

Still relating that operating costs tend to be lesser in comparison to centralized computer systems, varying according to the application, however, the distributed model involves sharing of storage and processing resources (Crosby et al. 2016, Drescher 2017, Zheng et al. 2017).

The requirement for a large processing capacity or a network capable of handling large volumes of data, which can be achieved through cloud computing, involves cryptographic procedures; a system of the type very accessed or with many nodes has high chances of overload (Crosby et al. 2016, Drescher 2017, Zheng et al. 2017).

To keep the system running smoothly, it may be necessary to spend financially on computers that support operations or on network equipment capable of supporting heavy data traffic, or invest in cloud computing platforms (Tasatanattakool & Techapanupreeda 2018, Applebaum et al. 2017, Kaushik et al. 2017).

In addition, depending on how the blockchain is structured, the response time for certain operations can be long, a situation that tends to cause considerable bottlenecks if the demand for use of the system increases, i.e., depending on the application, the operational cost of the system. Blockchain can also be elevated (Prusty 2017, Weber 2018, Crosby et al. 2016, Drescher 2017).

Several scenarios must be considered to prevent bottlenecks, decreased efficiency, or even security problems, which is why the development and deployment must be well planned (Applebaum et al. 2017, Kaushik et al. 2017, Zheng et al. 2017, Babkin et al. 2018, Idrees et al. 2021b).

Therefore, it is important that a thorough study should be carried out to assess whether the technology is a good solution for a particular application. Assessing criteria "such as" ensuring that there are no outages, under "what circumstances" it may be necessary to increase the capacity of the system, "which" procedures need to be adopted to prevent technology from breaching regulations or laws, and so on (Applebaum et al. 2017, Kaushik et al. 2017, Zheng et al. 2017, Babkin et al. 2018).

3.6   BLOCKCHAIN APPLICATIONS

Precisely the management of private records is the main interest of doctors and hospital managers, who will be able to exchange patient information with complete security and speed through digital means. Also related to the B2C (Business-to-consumer) relationship (companies for end customers), i.e., from doctors to patients, creating a relationship can be intensified in which the patient trusts the system and offers his personal and health data, feeding the health institution's big data directly, creating a history that can be recovered in times of illness or even to make diagnoses and anticipate treatments in certain groups of patients (Golosova & Romanovs 2018, Grover et al. 2018).

In health, with the availability of data on patients on a shared network, it can positively impact global health, assessing that a patient who begins treatment in another state or country can have all their examinations and histories transited in a digitally safe way, without edits or losses in the information. Likewise, the exchange of experiences among doctors with the studies of global diseases, forms of diagnosis, and treatment can be decentralized, creating big data of global health. Relating which diseases are most common in certain regions of the world, which medications are most used, stock control of the work material needed for treatments, among other information that is important to be shared, can transit via blockchain (Linn & Koo 2016, Golosova & Romanovs 2018, Grover et al. 2018).

Blockchain due to the characteristics of a distributed registry, data validation, can provide support for a more secure, universally accessible, and comprehensive health record system. Given that currently, a patient's medical history is a puzzle with its pieces spread by several suppliers and health organizations (Linn & Koo 2016, Golosova & Romanovs 2018, Grover et al. 2018).

Blockchain is possible to help put all these pieces together in real time and visualize the entire health context of a patient with the confidence of knowing that they are comprehensive and up-to-date, and digitally secure. This worldwide, highly distributed and secure access to patient data can provide authentic and universal access to patient medical records anywhere in the world (Linn & Koo 2016, Kuo et al. 2017, Grover et al. 2018).

Allowing medical requirements to be processed in a matter of seconds instead of weeks or months, also being able to "validate the supply chain," with respect to the time when a doctor writes a prescription, it is registered on the blockchain with a fair price for the consumer with major implications for order management for medical supplies and medicines (Linn & Koo 2016, Kuo et al. 2017, Angraal et al. 2017).

The health sector can employ blockchain to register recipes, conduct scientific research, and, consequently, reduce bureaucracy and logistical problems. Since medicine laboratories will be able to control all patients who have taken their substance and the most common supposed side effects, allowing research to be more detailed. Consequently, problems related to the supply of counterfeit drugs, through the chain of blocks, can identify the counterfeit product and reject it, preventing fraud (Linn & Koo 2016, Kuo et al. 2017, Angraal et al. 2017).

Blockchain could bring more transparency and organization to the pharmaceutical sector, reducing human problems and errors, relating that clinical tests may have more integrity of the data generated, maintaining patient privacy, and easier to interpret information. Through an integrated information network, the doctor, the laboratory, the pharmacist, the hospital, and the health plan will be able to obtain data on medical records in a decentralized, organized, and safe way (Linn & Koo 2016, Kuo et al. 2017, Angraal et al. 2017, Zhao et al. 2018).

Blockchain can also be used on a distributed network of digital transaction processors that handle sensitive clinical data for the healthcare industry, with the goal of providing a secure network for all sources of patient data. Thus, identity information, electronic medical record, in addition to medical devices, and interconnection between pharmacies, can perform a digital security eligibility check (Angraal et al. 2017, Zhao et al. 2018, Peterson et al. 2016).

Through the use of blockchain, it is possible to create an open-source database, in which health professionals access patient information and coordinate care more quickly. Using blockchain encryption, it speeds up care, automates administrative processes, creates smart contracts between patients and doctors, and also accesses data via mobile with total security (Linn & Koo 2016, Kuo et al. 2017, Mettler 2016).

Blockchain can also change the way healthcare services, in general, are priced and paid, due to improved identity management, smart contracts, and instant communication between machines enabled by the blockchain (Linn & Koo 2016, Kuo et al. 2017, Mettler 2016).

3.7 TRENDS

Using blockchain, tokenization of an asset transforms a digital fraction (token) of a digital contract, a property, a work of art, or even part of a company, is issued and the document represents a real asset. This fraction (token) has market value and can be negotiated quickly, with less bureaucracy and legal validation. Through digital tokenization, a company can raise funds by transferring a digital asset of nominal value to the owner within a smart contract. Still pondering that with the growth and appreciation of this company, your token can be traded within the company itself or with another investor, similar to what happens on the stock exchange, but more simply and inclusively (Oliveira et al. 2018, Westerkamp et al. 2020).

The use of the blockchain ensures that the data collected by smart devices (IoT) is not altered, given that the data collection associated with the blockchain, it is possible to ensure that the information is not altered due to its decentralized operation through encryption (Mazzei et al. 2020, Singh et al. 2020).

Based on the premise that blockchain depends on the collaboration of several parties, this is dependent on interconnectivity, which can be achieved through hybrid or even multi-cloud. The multi-cloud and hybrid cloud character will allow all actors in the chain to select the blockchain platform without depending on the infrastructure on which their data is hosted. Blockchain allows the ease of use of everything that healthcare companies need, in hybrid cloud, multi-cloud, and local environments, given the potential of the technology in which tens, hundreds, or even thousands of participants in a network (Yang et al. 2020, Aral et al. 2020).

Through blockchain, it is possible to capture millions of data points and spread across the world, relating adjacent technologies such as 5G, artificial intelligence (AI), and edge computing, which can be combined with blockchain generating added value for network participants. For example, the most reliable blockchain data will inform better, generate insights, and strengthen intelligent and machine learning algorithms (Rathi et al. 2020, Singh et al. 2020).

Or even through the greater adoption of blockchain and its characteristics, digital governance will become a key factor, making it possible to create a pragmatic governance model in which all participants agree. In fact, some health organizations still lack uniform digital governance standards among partners, in this respect, the advance in proof of concept (PoC) or the admission of a minimum viable ecosystem (MVE), which is when multiple stakeholders are able to exchange assets consistently, and not just test transactions on a platform (Satamraju 2020, Giraldo et al. 2020).

Although relatively immature, blockchain technology in health care is slowly starting to migrate from the proof of concept (PoC) that is used to verify that the technology works at a basic level, without even thinking about how it will actually perform in the market, i.e., it is a documented evidence that it can be successful, making it possible to identify technical errors that may interfere with the operation and expected results. And reaching the business-to-business (B2B) commercial, demonstrating the initial return on investments (ROIs) in initiatives focused on enterprise-level B2B, creating the much-needed network effect in the healthcare space (Hasselgren et al. 2020, Hanssen Rensaa et al. 2020).

3.8 DISCUSSION

The difficulty in breaking into a blockchain structure is related to the premise that when trying to delete a transaction that is inserted in a given block, a digital attacker would have to delete the transaction for that particular block and still control most of all computers on the network, that is, the network consensus (formed by thousands of people and has gigantic computational power), and discover the hashes of the next blocks.

It is also worth mentioning that he must do all this in minutes, which is the time for the next block to be formed, because the bigger this chain of blocks gets, the smaller the chances of a cyberattack becoming successful. Thus, the attacker could not simply modify information on the blockchain without controlling the majority of the network.

After all, to access the information contained in a block, it will be necessary to decipher the encryption of his hash and also of the previous block. As everything is connected like a chain, this process would have to be done successively and it would practically have no end. In addition, it would be necessary to change the data recorded on each of the various computers connected to the network, requiring that the cybercriminal's computer has a processing capacity greater than the total of all computers on the network.

The possibility of having an extremely secure database with complete information makes the blockchain extremely attractive to healthcare institutions that deal with sensitive data from patients who need to maintain permanent and reliable records.

The blocks are information registered in the blockchain are the transactions, which receive a confirmation from the network after the block in which they are inserted is mined, forming a hash compatible with that of the previous block. In this context, a cybercriminal finding a certain hash requires a high frequency of calculations, and this is very difficult. Because to perform this task, it requires thousands of calculations quickly, that is, a computer with extremely high processing power.

In this exemplified scenario, there is a high cost to digitally attack a blockchain where many computers cooperate, in such a way that the damage would be so great that the person who wishes to attack the network would probably prefer to cooperate with it to earn a greater reward.

Still relating that blockchain is not applicable in all situations and businesses, it is generally ideal for sales of non-falsifiable tickets, land registration, identity registration (through an online platform that allows the registration of documents and identity), and contracts (i.e., smart contracts between two people, without the need for an intermediary, through an online notary based on blockchain). Or even relating the modernity of social networks based on blockchain guaranteeing the freedom of expression of its users, or even authentication of documents, product tracking, carbon credits, school transcripts, diplomas, passports, car registrations, property registries, and among others. Other derivative branches, also use this technology through a blockchain-based digital wallet buying bitcoin cryptocurrencies. Still, this type of technology is appropriate for those healthcare corporations that require to record data transparently and reliably, such as medical records.

3.9 CONCLUSIONS

Blockchain is a distributed system that permits to track the receiving and sending of various kinds of information and data over the Internet; this is defined as a decentralized network marking the time of virtual transactions, placing it in a continuous chain in association with "hashes," composing a record without the possibility changes, i.e., without redoing all the work. The use of blockchain in health appears as a great ally of managers and professionals in the area, in times where the concern about data leakage grows exponentially, even more after the publication of the General Law for the Protection of Personal Data (LGPD) in several countries.

As the network is not centralized anywhere and has several layers of security, hacking is extremely difficult; it is the characteristic that makes blockchain a secure technology. When the system recognizes that someone is trying to break in, it automatically locks in a matter of seconds.

For not allowing data corruption and removing intermediaries from the information validation process, or even certification and authenticity of documents, registration of contracts, and intellectual property, the health-tech market must insert the blockchain in the healthcare sector as solutions from data storage systems, where doctors can maintain their professional and academic portfolio, or for hospitals to handle patient and staff data with complete security.

Still it is reflecting that there is a multitude of blockchain options for individuals and companies in various sectors, in addition to health care. Even considering the types of private, public, consortium, and even semiprivate blockchains, having many specifications, that provide different experiences that depending on the use, users will select the most suitable for their goals.

In summary, health institutions, doctors, health posts, and other institutions are starting to increase, making the blockchain even more accessible, seeing its full technological potential. Given the ability to sensibly protect a large amount of data, it is one of the main benefits of using blockchain in health. In addition, as it has a decentralized and transparent nature, this technology also enables the sharing of information between health professionals and patients quickly and safely.

Finally, it is possible to state that the future of tools such as blockchain for health care is very promising, since this structure has the potential to support a rigorous system for preserving patient data and, at the same time, expand access to information on new discoveries and scientific studies.

REFERENCES

Angraal, S., Krumholz, H. M., & Schulz, W. L. (2017). Blockchain technology: Applications in health care. *Circulation: Cardiovascular Quality and Outcomes*, 10(9), e003800.

Applebaum, B., Haramaty-Krasne, N., Ishai, Y., Kushilevitz, E., & Vaikuntanathan, V. (2017). Low-complexity cryptographic hash functions. *In 8th Innovations in Theoretical Computer Science Conference (ITCS 2017). Schloss Dagstuhl-Leibniz-Zentrum fuer Informatik.* University of California at Berkeley

Aral, A., Uriarte, R. B., Simonet-Boulogne, A., & Brandic, I. (2020, May). Reliability management for blockchain-based decentralized multi-cloud. *In 2020 20th IEEE/ACM International Symposium on Cluster, Cloud, and Internet Computing (CCGRID)*, (pp. 21–30). IEEE. Melbourne, Australia

Babkin, A. V., Burkaltseva, D. D., Betskov, A. V., Kilyaskhanov, H. S., Tyulin, A. S., & Kurianova, I. V. (2018). Automation digitalization blockchain: Trends and implementation problems. *International Journal of Engineering and Technology (UAE)*, 7(3.14 Special Issue 14), 254–260.

Biswas, K., & Muthukkumarasamy, V. (2016, December). Securing smart cities using blockchain technology. In 2016 IEEE 18th International Conference on High-Performance Computing and Communications; IEEE *14th* International Conference on Smart City; IEEE *2nd* International Conference on Data Science and Systems (HPCC/SmartCity/DSS), (pp. 1392–1393). IEEE: Sydney, NSW.

Cachin, C., & Vukolić, M. (2017). Blockchain consensus protocols in the wild. arXiv preprint arXiv:1707.01873.

Crosby, M., Pattanayak, P., Verma, S., & Kalyanaraman, V. (2016). Blockchain technology: Beyond bitcoin. *Applied Innovation*, 2(6–10), 71.

Drescher, D. (2017). *Blockchain Basics* (Vol. 276). Berkeley, CA: Apress.

Gabison, G. (2016). Policy considerations for the blockchain technology public and private applications. *SMU Science & Technology Law Review*, 19, 327.

Gervais, A., Karame, G. O., Wüst, K., Glykantzis, V., Ritzdorf, H., & Capkun, S. (2016, October). On the security and performance of proof of work blockchains. *In Proceedings of the 2016 ACM SIGSAC Conference on Computer and Communications Security* (pp. 3–16).

Giraldo, F. D., Barbosa, M. C., & Gamboa, C. E. (2020). Electronic voting using blockchain and smart contracts: Proof of concept. *IEEE Latin America Transactions*, 100, 1e.

Golosova, J., & Romanovs, A. (2018, November). The advantages and disadvantages of the blockchain technology. *In 2018 IEEE 6th Workshop on Advances in Information, Electronic and Electrical Engineering (AIEEE)*, (pp. 1–6). IEEE. Vilnius, Lithuania

Grover, P., Kar, A. K., & Ilavarasan, P. V. (2018, October). Blockchain for businesses: A systematic literature review. *In Conference on e-Business, e-Services, and e-Society*, (pp. 325–336). Springer, Cham. Kuwait City, Kuwait

Gupta, S. S. (2017). *Blockchain*. Hoboken, NJ: John Wiley & Sons, Inc.

Gupta, S., & Sadoghi, M. (2019). Blockchain transaction processing.

Hakak, S., Khan, W. Z., Gilkar, G. A., Imran, M., & Guizani, N. (2020). Securing smart cities through blockchain technology: Architecture, requirements, and challenges. *IEEE Network*, 34(1), 8–14.

Hanssen Rensaa, J. A., Gligoroski, D., Kralevska, K., Hasselgren, A., & Faxvaag, A. (2020). VerifyMed--A blockchain platform for transparent trust in virtualized healthcare: Proof-of-concept. arXiv, arXiv-2005.

Hasselgren, A., Kralevska, K., Gligoroski, D., Pedersen, S. A., & Faxvaag, A. (2020). Blockchain in healthcare and health sciences: A scoping review. *International Journal of Medical Informatics*, 134, 104040.

Idrees, S. M., Nowostawski, M., & Jameel, R. (2021a). Blockchain-based digital contact tracing apps for COVID-19 pandemic management: Issues, challenges, solutions, and future directions. *JMIR Medical Informatics*, 9(2), e25245.

Idrees, S.M.; Nowostawski, M.; Jameel, R.; Mourya, A.K. Security Aspects of Blockchain Technology Intended for Industrial Applications. Electronics 2021, 10, 951. https://doi.org/10.3390/electronics10080951

Idrees, S. M., Nowostawski, M., Jameel, R., & Mourya, A. K. (2021b). Privacy-preserving. In: P. Churi, A. Pawar, & A. A. Elngar (Eds), *Data Protection and Privacy in Healthcare: Research and Innovations* (p. 109). CRC Press, Boca Raton, FL.

Jiang, S., & Wu, J. (2020, October). A game-theoretic approach to storage offloading in PoC-based mobile blockchain mining. *In Proceedings of the Twenty-First International Symposium on Theory, Algorithmic Foundations, and Protocol Design for Mobile Networks and Mobile Computing*, (pp. 171–180).

Kaushik, A., Choudhary, A., Ektare, C., Thomas, D., & Akram, S. (2017, May). Blockchain: Literature survey. *In 2017 2nd IEEE International Conference on Recent Trends in Electronics, Information & Communication Technology (RTEICT)*, (pp. 2145–2148). IEEE. Bangalore, India

Kim, S., Kwon, Y., & Cho, S. (2018, October). A survey of scalability solutions on blockchain. *In 2018 International Conference on Information and Communication Technology Convergence (ICTC),* (pp. 1204–1207). IEEE. Jeju Island, Korea,

Kuo, T. T., Kim, H. E., & Ohno-Machado, L. (2017). Blockchain distributed ledger technologies for biomedical and health care applications. *Journal of the American Medical Informatics Association,* 24(6), 1211–1220.

Li, W., Andreina, S., Bohli, J. M., & Karame, G. (2017). Securing proof-of-stake blockchain protocols. *In Data Privacy Management, Cryptocurrencies, and Blockchain Technology* (pp. 297–315). Springer, Cham.

Linn, L. A., & Koo, M. B. (2016). Blockchain for health data and its potential use in health it and healthcare-related research. *In ONC/NIST Use of Blockchain for Healthcare and Research Workshop,* Gaithersburg, Maryland, ONC/NIST, (pp. 1–10).

Lu, Y. (2018). Blockchain and the related issues: A review of current research topics. *Journal of Management Analytics,* 5(4), 231–255.

Mazzei, D., Baldi, G., Fantoni, G., Montelisciani, G., Pitasi, A., Ricci, L., & Rizzello, L. (2020). A blockchain Tokenizer for industrial IOT trustless applications. *Future Generation Computer Systems,* 105, 432–445.

Mengelkamp, E., Notheisen, B., Beer, C., Dauer, D., & Weinhardt, C. (2018). A blockchain-based smart grid: towards sustainable local energy markets. *Computer Science-Research and Development,* 33(1–2), 207–214.

Mettler, M. (2016, September). Blockchain technology in healthcare: The revolution starts here. *In 2016 IEEE 18th International Conference on e-Health Networking, Applications, and Services (Healthcom),* (pp. 1–3). IEEE. Munich, Germany

Oliveira, L., Zavolokina, L., Bauer, I., & Schwabe, G. (2018). To token or not to token: Tools for understanding blockchain tokens.

Peterson, K., Deeduvanu, R., Kanjamala, P., & Boles, K. (2016, September). A blockchain-based approach to health information exchange networks. *In Proceedings of NIST Workshop Blockchain Healthcare,* (Vol. 1, No. 1, pp. 1–10).

Prusty, N. (2017). *Building Blockchain Projects.* Birmingham: Packt Publishing Ltd.

Rathi, V. K., Chaudhary, V., Rajput, N. K., Ahuja, B., Jaiswal, A. K., Gupta, D., ... & Hammoudeh, M. (2020). A blockchain-enabled multi-domain edge computing orchestrator. *IEEE Internet of Things Magazine,* 3(2), 30–36.

Satamraju, K. P. (2020). Proof of concept of scalable integration of internet of things and blockchain in healthcare. *Sensors,* 20(5), 1389.

Singh, S. K., Rathore, S., & Park, J. H. (2020). Blockiotintelligence: A blockchain-enabled intelligent IoT architecture with artificial intelligence. *Future Generation Computer Systems,* 110, 721–743.

Tasatanattakool, P., & Techapanupreeda, C. (2018, January). Blockchain: Challenges and applications. *In 2018 International Conference on Information Networking (ICOIN),* (pp. 473–475). IEEE. Chiang Mai, Thailand

Van Rijmenam, M., & Ryan, P. (2018). *Blockchain: Transforming Your Business and Our World.* London: Routledge.

Wang, W., Hoang, D. T., Xiong, Z., Niyato, D., Wang, P., Hu, P., & Wen, Y. (2018). A survey on consensus mechanisms and mining management in blockchain networks. arXiv preprint arXiv:1805.02707, 1–33.

Weber, R. M. (2018). An advisor's introduction to blockchain. *Journal of Financial Service Professionals,* 72(6), 49–53.

Westerkamp, M., Victor, F., & Küpper, A. (2020). Tracing manufacturing processes using blockchain-based token compositions. *Digital Communications and Networks,* 6(2), 167–176.

Xu, X., Weber, I., & Staples, M. (2019). *Architecture for Blockchain Applications* (pp. 1–307). Heidelberg: Springer.

Yang, X., Pei, X., Wang, M., Li, T., & Wang, C. (2020). Multi-replica and multi-cloud data public audit scheme based on blockchain. *IEEE Access*, 8, 144809–144822.

Zhao, D. (2020). Cross-blockchain transactions. *In Conference on Innovative Data Systems Research (CIDR)*. Amsterdam, Netherlands

Zhao, H., Bai, P., Peng, Y., & Xu, R. (2018). Efficient key management scheme for health blockchain. *CAAI Transactions on Intelligence Technology*, 3(2), 114–118.

Zheng, Z., Xie, S., Dai, H., Chen, X., & Wang, H. (2017, June). An overview of blockchain technology: Architecture, consensus, and future trends. In *2017 IEEE International Congress on Big Data (BigData Congress)*, (pp. 557–564). IEEE. Boston, MA, USA

4 Blockchain Technology: A Panacea for Medical Distribution Ailments

Richa Chauhan
Banasthali Vidyapith

Vidhi Kaul
Independent Researcher

CONTENTS

4.1 INTRODUCTION

Since the last decade, academician and industry people have been attracted toward blockchain technology (Michael et al., 2018). It is recognized as a technology of distributed ledger, which facilitates peer-to-peer (P2P) network of digital data transactions. This network of digital data transactions may be privately or publicly dispersed among all concerned users, and in turn permitting the storage of all types of digital data transactions in an authentic and testable manner (Gaggioli, 2018). Smart contract is another prominent notion of blockchain technology, which comprises of a tailor-made set of regulations, under whose supervision various stakeholders willingly interact in the non-centralized, atomized format. Innumerable applications of smart contract have risen in various sectors, ranging from financial services to energy resources, from healthcare to voting (Macrinici et al., 2018). Blockchain technology puts forward lucidity and obliterates the requirement of third-party officials or arbitrators (Pilkington, 2016). In an erratic business environment, blockchain technology uses the procedure of consensus and the technique of cryptography to test the authenticity of a transaction (Yang et al., 2019). In a dispersed peer-to-peer network of digital data transactions of blockchain technology, messages are verified by accepted nodes; if the received messages are accurate, then only they get stored in a block. In order to affirm the data stored in each block, consensus theorem is utilized; this consensus theorem or algorithm is known by the name "Proof-of-Work". Then the verified block shall be annexed into the chain, and each node in the network of digital data transactions acknowledges the respective block and the chain expands ceaselessly (Lin & Liao, 2017) (Figure 4.1).

4.2   CATEGORIES OF BLOCKCHAIN STRUCTURES

There are mainly four categories of blockchain setup namely: public, private, consortium, and hybrid blockchains (Hölbl et al., 2018).

- **Public Blockchains**: Completely non-centralized network of data is facilitated by public blockchains. This is an application where each stakeholder can retrieve the data and can also participate in the process of consensus (e.g., Bitcoin and Ethereum) (Alhadhrami et al., 2017).
- **Private Blockchains**: Private blockchains facilitates are dedicated solutions to one company only. Further, it promotes audit of alteration of data happening between various individual officials and departments of the same. Each and every contributor requires permission to become a part of the network and to be called as a member or a stakeholder once the consent is received (Choi, 2020).
- **Consortium Blockchains**: Consortium blockchain is a restricted network of data transactions, and it is public only for a few people or groups. Consortium blockchain is used to supervise and audit alterations of dispersed data among respective members.
- **Hybrid Blockchains**: Hybrid blockchains incorporates the merits of public and private blockchains. That is why, public blockchains utilized to prepare ledgers which are completely retrievable, whereas private blockchain keeps on operating in the background so as to restrict the retrieval of changes in the ledger (Qiao et al., 2018) (Figure 4.2).

4.3   BLOCKCHAIN AND HEALTH CARE
INDUSTRY (BACKGROUND)

Healthcare industry is one of the major sectors or industry, where blockchain technology can be applied efficiently and effectively and could also result in countering issues with respect to sharing and storing of data, its security, and privacy (Kshetri, 2017). The

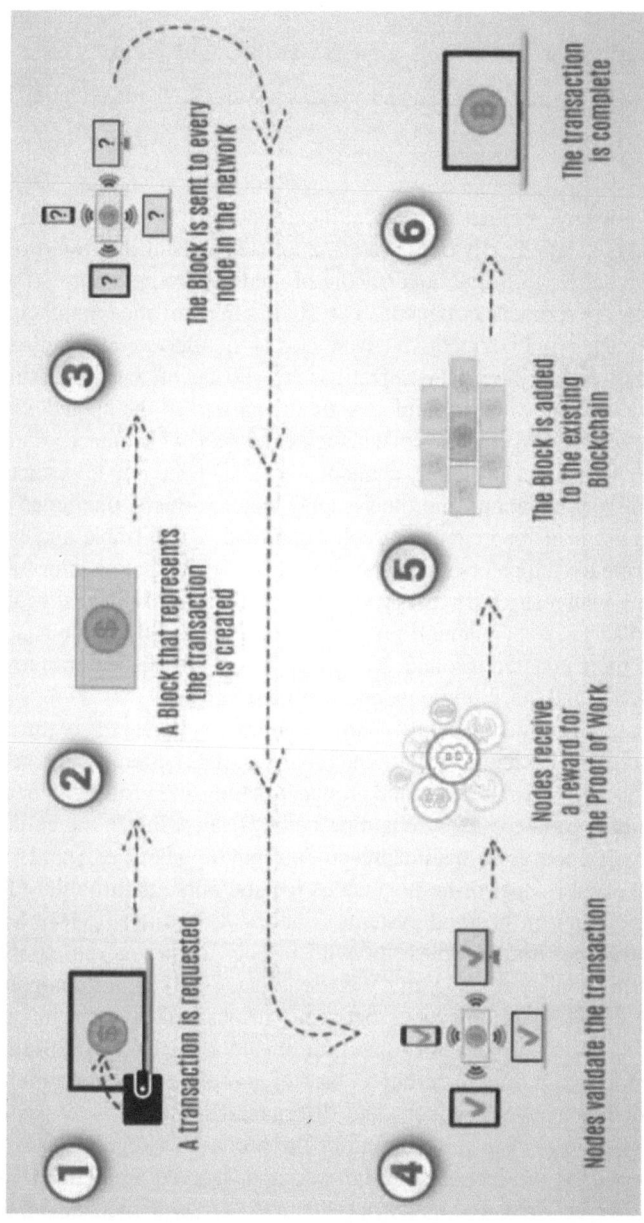

FIGURE 4.1 Blockchain architecture diagram. (Source: https://datascience.foundation/sciencewhitepaper/top-5-use-cases-and-platforms-of-block-chain-technology.)

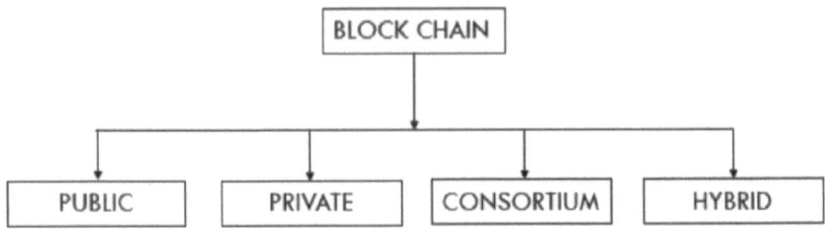

FIGURE 4.2   Categories of blockchain.

biggest expenditure seeking area in the health care industry is supply chain management (SCM) and concerned activities (Scalise, 2005). The healthcare SCM operations broadly comprise delivery on time and tracing of medical products across the system until it reaches the concerned user/patients. Past studies in retail and manufacturing had quantified the strategic and competitive advantages of an effective and well-organized SCM, but healthcare contributing organizations are still far off from encashing these advantages. Various deprecatory roadblocks are recognized in the application of well organized and efficient SCM solutions in healthcare industry, which incorporates lack of proper education with respect to supply chain matters and underlying misunderstanding among purchasing organizations and other supply chain partners, unaligned financial motivations, requirement for better data collection, and recognizable and well-organized key performance indicators (McKone-Sweet, 2005). Ineffective information systems and software with restricted synergy aggravate the drawbacks in healthcare supply chain. Present disorganized, manual, and impromptu practices for medical product traceability give more concrete ground to come up with a compelling case to embrace artificial intelligence and machine-bounded learning solutions.

A large number of healthcare supply chain literature accentuate the requirement for more and more organized electronic data interchange (EDI) systems and consolidated information technology (IT) for upgraded product tracking and visibility. For example, implementation of organized supply chain procedures can result in the enhancement of quality and cost controls in healthcare product buying (Ford & Scanlon, 2006). There is a necessity for superior homogeneous logistic pursuits through redesigning and work-based costing in hospital systems (Landry & Philippe, 2004). Moreover, there are several issues and complexities with respect to the internal supply chain management of hospital systems (Landry & Beaulieu, 2013). Non-homogeneity and the presence of non-aligned objectives between various stakeholders in healthcare industry adversely influence decisions based on inventory (De Vries, 2011). Various issues are dependency on human resource, lack of coordination among main player, vulnerable order management process and disorganized warehouse inventory, loss of information with respect to the demand of the product on regular basis, temperature variations during product transit and warehousing, requirement for shipment traceability, insufficient data, and inappropriate product tracing mechanism to curtail expiry and shortage of the product (Privett & Gonsalvez, 2014).

Today, compatibility and network inefficiencies, along with the nonavailability of platform for the purpose of authentic and viable data exchange, have given birth to the requirement with respect to a technique that could improvise the function of collecting, storing, and sharing viable data among various systems and stakeholders. The ever-increasing price of medicines and healthcare services makes the adoption of technologies and innovative measures to counter these complexities a must activity. Activities and processes in healthcare supply chain which require effective systems are keeping track of product expiry, product recalls, effective tracking system to trace shortages, and spurious or counterfeit drugs. These activities and processes are very lengthy and become cumbersome due to the absence of visibility and non-integrated and siloed logistics and on the top of that numerous stakeholders are engaged in overseeing healthcare supply chain processes (Chang et al., 2019).

SCM is structured to incorporate the latest techniques of industries with an objective to streamline the complete delivery methods starting from order to the supply of the product (Lee et al., 2011). Prospects of healthcare supply chain are very challenging; with disintegrated ordering patterns of medical supplies as well as availability of key critical resources and drugs, there is always an intrinsic risk of compromised supply chain procedure that might adversely impact patients' life (Kim & Kim, 2019). Survey of the World Health Organization (WHO) reveals that inappropriate dosage of counterfeited drugs ordered from unknown vendors and distributors was responsible for the death of not <100,000 people in Africa alone (World Health Organisation, 2017). Furthermore, not only the spurious product and drug whereas product registration and improper and non-fulfillment of packaging standards in a healthcare sector result in the disruption of the overall supply chain management (Jayaraman et al., 2018). Blockchain technology is specifically an auditing system that monitors the entire process of medical products and drugs evolution (Dujak & Sajter, 2019). Blockchain technology facilitates instant identification and viability of not only the origin of the drug but also of its vendor and the distributor, as there is an entry of each and every transaction onto the digital ledger. Blockchain maintains systematic record of every node. Moreover, this distributed digitalized ledger also permits doctors, physicians, and healthcare officials to review and validate the recommendations of suppliers (Narayanaswami et al., 2019). Better understanding of the supply chain procedure via genuine and prompt validation process leads healthcare providers and pharmacies toward obstacle-free delivery of authentic drugs to those patients who are in need of them the most. Blockchain technology facilitates establishment of a very credible and dependable network of distributors and vendors that authorize healthcare administrators to protect patients from suppliers of infamous and notorious repute. Further, blockchain technology plays a vital role in the increment of authentic sources of data, forecasting of demand, avoidance of fraud, and digitized transactions (Funk et al., 2018).

4.4   PROCESS OF MEDICAL SUPPLY CHAIN IN BLOCKCHAIN

Step 1: As soon as new medicine is developed which incorporates patent rights and a lengthy procedure of clinical trials, a specific block is generated. Now this block records all information with respect to the clinical trials and process details in a form of digital ledger transactions.

Step 2: When clinical trials achieve success, manufacturing unit will receive patent for prototype testing and mass manufacturing, and each and every clinically approved medicine or product will receive its unique recognition, which in turn will be amalgamated with another block in the respective blockchain incorporating other important information about the product.

Step 3: As soon as the mass production and packaging activity is completed, medicines are sent to the warehouse for distribution in future. Blockchain incorporates several information like barcode, date and time of manufacture, lot identification number, and date of expiry.

Step 4: Blockchain may incorporate transportation details like time of dispatch from one warehouse (out) to the receiving time (IN) to the other, transportation mode, name of authorized agent, and many more.

Step 5: Healthcare providers or retailers receive drugs and medical supplies generally through a third-party distribution network. A warehouse (OUT) for each third party is used for this purpose from where all distribution endpoints are linked. A separate transaction is also integrated into the blockchain.

Step 6: Healthcare providers, for example, clinics or hospitals, are required to generate information like name of owner of the product, lot number, batch number, date of expiry to validate authenticity of the drug and in turn prevent counterfeit. These information are also incorporated in the blockchain.

Step 7: Blockchain supply chain serves verifiable and transparent information to potential buyers, and patients are motivated to check the authenticity and validity of the product throughout the complete process (Bocek et al., 2017).

4.4.1 CLINICAL TRIALS

Clinical trials in healthcare industry incorporate many challenges and complexities which include privacy of personal data, sharing of data, and patient enrolment (Isojarvi et al., 2018). The technology which can successfully address all these complexities and many more is blockchain. Blockchain furnishes several models for the exchange of clinical trial information which enhances the transparency and reproduction of data in a secured environment (Benchoufi et al., 2017; Idrees et al. 2021). Smart contracts technology namely Ethereum which work on a private network can be proposed to counter degradation of trust among stakeholders and underprop transparency of data in clinical trials. With the purpose of increasing the potentiality of clinical trials and fidelity of medicines, four more new structures have been evolved in addition to the traditional blockchain technology (Nugent et al., 2016).

These new structures or systems comprises of blockchain-based distribution aligned computing model for big data analytics; data management system for the integration of data; identification management system for protection of privacy on Internet of Things (IoT) devices; and data exchange management system for purpose of research collaboration (Shae & Tsai, 2017). Novel data management structure which is permission-based blockchain technology utilizing smart contract is also advisable (Choudhury et al., 2019). The main objective of this proposed technology was to come up with a mechanism that could reduce the time, burden of administrative activities, and the pain of securing integrity and privacy of data in a multilevel clinical trials approach. Consent workflow system was also developed with the

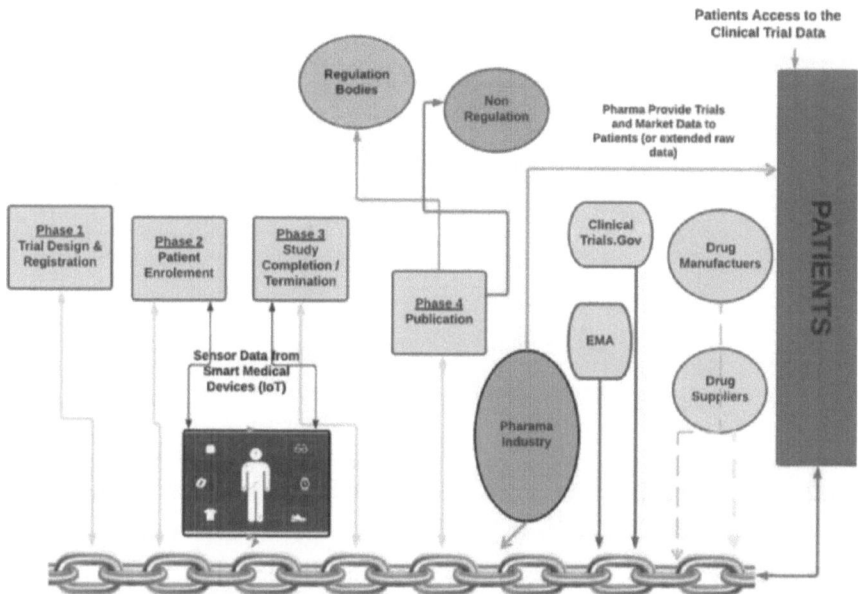

FIGURE 4.3 Ethereum blockchain for clinical trials. (Source: https://link.springer.com/chapter/10.1007/978-3-030-11289-9_3.)

clinical trial method. This system is a proof-of-concept arrangement of blockchain technology, and it is relied on the collection of consent on the basis of time stamping, including the accession of smart contract. Consent workflow system is competent in imparting transparency and conformity to an extremely sensitive data, even when the data is recorded public website (Benchouf & Ravaud, 2017) (Figure 4.3).

4.4.2 Pharmaceutical

Pharmaceutical companies are persistent in not only coming up with the improvised version of medicines with respect to their quality and usability but at the same time trying to develop and innovate new medicines for various diseases. These relentless efforts of pharmaceutical companies are neither easy nor can be completed in less time; moreover, the entire process is highly complex and cumbersome comprising of many activities namely ensuring protection of patent, acquiescence by regulatory and administering bodies, safety, security, effectiveness and statistical viability of the data, transactions, and relevant information. In general, such processes are very time taking as they start with inventions and end with the commercialized use of medicines or products (Schöner et al., 2017).

Furthermore, such lengthy processes lead to spurious and counterfeit medicines as well as problems in medicine recall due to lack of safety and privacy of data (Marucheck et al., 2011). Blockchain technology can be a solution to these hurdles and could facilitate the removal of such complexities throughout the process of pharmaceutical sector. Blockchains use distributed ledger which could enhance privacy

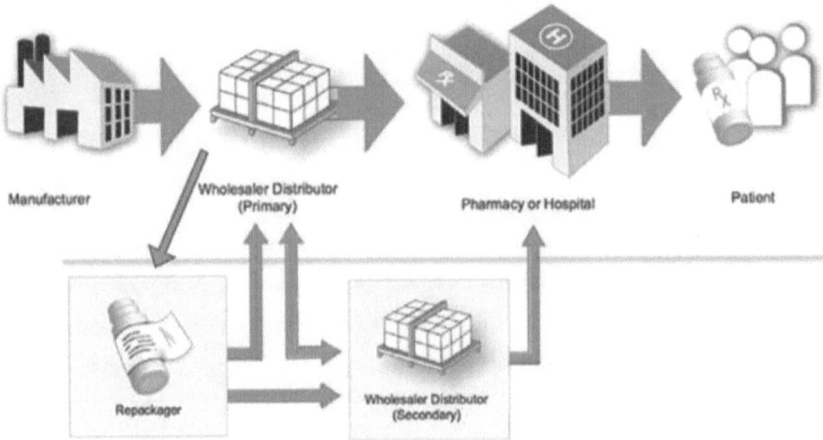

Manufacturer   Wholesaler Distributor   Pharmacy or Hospital   Patient
                          (Primary)

Repackager   Wholesaler Distributor
                                             (Secondary)

FIGURE 4.4   Blockchain in pharma. (Source: https://www.pharmafocusasia.com/strategy/ blockchain-technology-pharmaceutical-industry.)

and establish reliability, as every trial with respect to medicine is documented in blockchain nodes which cannot be modified. A private blockchain enables patent protection and could be successfully used to establish that each and every pharmaceutical company adheres to it. This can be achieved through the utilization of a smart contract. Smart contracts are capable of providing solidarity, accountability, and lucidity (Westerkamp et al., 2019). As per the recent study, about 60% of pharmaceutical industry is engaged with blockchain either via working on it or experimenting with it, and this very much authenticates the prospective of blockchain for the same. Counterfeit drugs or medicines are a global challenge which poses a tremendous risk to the life of consumers or general public (Figure 4.4).[1]

Pharma co-surveillance blockchain system is developed to check the practical application of the technology in a surveillance system of pharmaceutical sector. The main objective was to improvise the efficiency to track spurious drugs. The system combats with standard drug supply chain forging which is one of the notable matters in Asian countries. In this context, Global Governance Coin plays a vital role in each of the nodes, including full or normal node in a pyramid relationship and coin issuer which are used in drug supply chain management (Sylim et al., 2018). Gcoin blockchain system works as a platform that ensures the flow of information of drugs to come up with more pellucid data of drug transaction. This data is made available among producers, wholesalers, retailers, pharmacies, hospitals, and consumers. Gcoin technology can successfully convert medicine supply chain from regulating activity to surveillance activity where every stakeholder from manufacturer to consumer is collaborating. Furthermore, the regulation structure of the medicine supply chain could be altered from the scrutiny and inspection to the surveillance network structure (Tseng et al., 2018). For more than a decade, radio frequency identification (RFID)

---

[1] 60 of Pharma Companies Using or Trying Blockchain Survey. Available online: https://pharmaphorum. com/news/60-of-pharma-companies-using-or-trying-blockchain-survey/.

technology has been contemplated to be a powerful technique for the protection of an owner; nevertheless, out of the trusted realm RFID, for example, the post supply chain network is often being forged due to its vulnerability by duplicating this identification. Ethereum system and its wallet are capable of removing such vulnerabilities throughout the complete supply chain system, beginning from producers to the end consumers (Toyoda et al., 2017).

4.4.3 Usability of Blockchain Technology in Claims of Supply Chain Management and Management of Medical Bills

The contribution of healthcare service to the whole healthcare industry is increasing rapidly, resulting in the worth a trillion dollars (Toyoda et al., 2017). Medical billing is one of the important segments of the healthcare sector, as without this process reliable and verifiable delivery of medical services are not possible. This process of medical billing starts at the time when a respective patient is admitted and until he or she checks out of the hospital. The process of medical billing comprises various activities namely checking-in, conformation with respect to financial obligation, complaisance of coding and billing formalities, and forwarding the claim and reception of payments from insurance companies.[2] The complete billing system becomes more complex and challenging when the health insurance plan of an individual patient covers the complete fees of the treatment. The excessive billing is one of the major concerns in the process of medical billing, as there is absence of clarity and transparency; furthermore, doctors lack trust among their own fraternity, insurance companies, and patients. In the healthcare sector, medical claims and billing process are often misused and exploited. Blockchain technology can minimize or completely solve the problem of exploitation of medical claims and bills by facilitating a very transparent system and abolishing the lack of trust among stakeholders engaged in the system (Deisingh, 2005).

4.4.3.1 Management of Quality

Counterfeit drugs are those which contain inappropriate elements or additives, and are consciously traded with an intention of imitating their radix, validity, or effectiveness (Zhu & Kouhizadeh, 2019). Furthermore, counterfeit drugs and medical products put an adverse impact on the viability of medical supply chain management (Plotnikov & Kuznetsova, 2018). Their performance in the pharmaceutical industry is competitive factor that disrupts the efficiency, authenticity, and robust profitability in a particular healthcare industry enormously. Globally consumers are vulnerable, as often they are unaware of the origin of the products they buy and consume (Montecchi et al., 2019). As counterfeit drugs are malicious, they not only pose a life-threatening risk to the patients around the world, but also a threat to the trustworthiness of the original pharmaceutical companies, drug manufacturers, and vendors, who keep on investing a huge volume of money on counteractants (Kumar et al., 2018). Techniques namely spectroscopic and chromatographic are very efficient in the identification of

---

[2] Course2: The Medical Billing Process. Available online: https://www.medicalbillingandcodingonline. com/medical-coding-for-billers/.

counterfeit elements as they can locate original elements and composition. However, these techniques are electromechanical apparatus bases which in turn increase the overhead cost. One of the very effective ways to solve these complexities successfully is to have product package number and serial numbers along with the pharmaceutical manufacturers' information, on the blockchain, from where drug manufacturers, pharmaceutical companies, and customers could authenticate and check the viability of the available data. Blockchain technology confirms registration of product, quality control at low cost, tracing of drug, and identification of counterfeit drug throughout the supply chain management process.[3]

4.4.4 INTERNET OF MEDICAL THINGS

Internet of medical things systems can contribute a lot in the evolution of information systems with respect to medicine, healthcare devices, and equipment. For example body scanners, wearable devices, heart monitors etc. can be arranged; orders can be processed; and relevant data and information can be shared over the Internet of Medical Things (IoMT) in no time (Chiuchisan et al., 2014). Expansion and innovations in artificial intelligence enable and promote healthcare providers to use the IoMT platform. With the help of this platform or technology, healthcare providers can take an image of the product, can identify faulty or spurious parts or dubious cells, and can share this piece of information or knowledge with another rightful stakeholder. The following steps explain the working of the IoMT.

Step 1: In the case of IoMT system of blockchain technology, all information and data are collected from patients.

Step 2: IoMT systems produce volumes of data through devices which are monitoring or observing patients' body either closely or from distance.

Step 3: Cloud storage or blocks are used to record data and information which are produced by IoMT systems. Then artificial intelligence is used to develop a virtual agent. Furthermore, a new ledger will be developed by this virtual agent automatically. Where medical data is highly sensitive and requires security in the first place, this artificial intelligence which is non-centralized in nature could generate a blockchain with the highest security.

Step 4: In the systems of IoMT, healthcare providers are the end consumers which always look forward for the careful, safe, and secured delivery of products from the system authorized by the owner (Moosavi et al., 2015).

4.4.5 HEALTHCARE IoT AND MEDICAL DEVICES

IoT is a congregation of online devices having unique identification with programmable capability to share data over internet without man-machine interchange. This capability makes IoT play a critical role in healthcare (Moosavi et al., 2015). Patient vitals monitoring medical devices are the core of IoMT (Haghi et al., 2017). People

---

[3] Decentralized AI: Blockchain's Bright Future. Available online: https://espeoblockchain.com/blog/decentralized-ai-benefits.

are using wearable IOT devices to monitor pulse, heart rate, blood pressure, calories burnt, and even remind them of time of medical examination or doctor appointments; this has been enabled due to a critical enabler called wireless body area network (WBAN) (Dimitrov, 2016). This chapter discusses a novel perspective on the integration of IoMT with blockchain. Griggs et al. (2018) introduced the integration of WBANs with blockchain smart contracts for uncompromised live patient monitoring and medical treatment. The study suggests running smart contracts in blockchain to examine and analyze information collected from patient's IoMT devices based on patient-specific value range of vitals. Rahman et al. (2018) introduced an intelligent dyslexia analytics solution that captured mobile multimedia health data during dyslexia testing which is stored on a big data repository over decentralized architecture to be shared with healthcare communities and individuals using blockchain for clinical research and statistical data analytics. Jo et al.(2018) using IoT and blockchain technology proposed a localized storage and globalized data distribution architecture by dividing it into edge and core networks. This enhanced the efficiency and adaptability of blockchain system. Zhang et al. (2016) conferred a model for the employment of attention supported a stable Policy Service Nodes (PSN). This model's primary challenge is to confirm the protection of data, once exchanging data or information between PSN nodes. The study developed two protocols to tackle this complication. The design of fundamental protocol is an upgraded version of IEEE802.15.6, which establishes stable ties with unbalanced procedural necessities for mobile devices and resource-limited sensor nodes, whereas the latter utilizes blockchain technology to allocate health data between PSN nodes. Ichikawa et al. (2017) developed a sabotage-proof mobile health system using blockchain technology to make a resilient record keeping. The objective of their study was to develop a mobile health database for cognitive behavioral therapy for insomnia patients using a smartphone application.

4.4.5.1   Healthcare IoT Infrastructure and Data Security

The infrastructure of Healthcare Information and Communication Technology comprises various IoT and network devices; for example, wireless access points, terminals, diagnostic machines, and sensor. This technical infrastructure facilitates systems of healthcare services namely remote monitoring services and instruments which are wearable to share and communicate critical information with respect to the condition of patients to caretakers. Throughout the process of transmission, data and information are very vulnerable and prone to privacy and safety breach. There are a number of incidents: for example, three phishing attacks cost breach of personal information of 20,000 patient's at Catawba Valley Medical Centre in North Carolina,[4] where attackers are trying to obtain any critical shortcoming to probe the healthcare network and arbitrate valuable data of service providers. In order to face the above-mentioned issues in healthcare IoT, analyst and researchers are trying to explore different techniques and technical methods, so that illegal penetration of user's data can be stopped. For example, Nikoloudakis et al. (2019) suggested a

---

[4] 3 Phishing Hacks Breach 20,000 Catawba Valley Patient Records. Available online: https://www. healthcareitnews.com/news/3-phishing-hacks-breach-20000-catawba-valley-patient-records (accessed on 20 April 2019).

software-defined network that virtualizes the traditional network infrastructure to determine a resistance mechanism against malevolent attacks at multiple extraction levels. The study introduced a fog computing design that uses the OpenVAS platform to check vulnerabilities of newly added and current hardware as well in healthcare IoT. The major challenge of the suggested model is the average time taken by a single device to assess the data is ~7 minutes and 21 seconds, which is just too long and poses serious questions about the system's quantifiability. Since block mining time is 10–15 seconds, this drawback may be resolved by the usage of blockchain-based Ethereum platform. Other research endeavors by Nausheen and Begum (2018) suggested a special approach for the safety of key logic and mobile applications, supported application hardening like code obfuscation and application program interface (APIs). The study advances the inclusion of a security layer through return-oriented programming via reverse engineering and check-summing techniques. However, the study properly addressed the protection of implanted medical gadgets and heterogeneous technologies required to enhance accumulative performance, but at the same time increases the complexity of the whole system. The study enforced Adaptively Supervised and Clustered Hybrid (ASCH-IDS) technology to boost the Intrusion Detection Systems (IDSs) in IoT networks, which categorize prospective intruders from collective sensory information or data. Varying proportion of collective sensory data traffic is fed into two detection subsystems: Anomaly Detection Systems (ADSs) and Misuse Detection Systems (MDSs) for higher performance. Curiously, the device performs well once the proportion amendment will increase, and it displays the best accuracy in terms of sensitivity and exactness once the proportion of sensory information on misuse detection is 0%:25%. This technique reveals increased and improved rate of detection. Furthermore, the study proposed (Catarinucci et al. 2015) the use of Restricted Boltzmann Machine-based Clustered IDS (RBC-IDS), a deep learning-based technique for observing critical and sensitive infrastructure for prospective intruders via three hidden layers that exhibit 99.91% higher accuracy compared to 99.80% in the previous report. The overhead price of this new experiment, however, is double the proposed model. Self-driven autonomous vehicles are now slowly and gradually shaping the present transportation system, and its application in healthcare sector is also indispensable, particularly in medical supply chain. Aloqaily et al. (2019) proposed a mechanism for intrusion identification and detection to resist denial of service, remote user, probe, etc. The study proposed a deep belief network for the reduction of knowledge dimensions and a choice tree for intrusion classification exploitation of the ID3 formula. The system's detection accuracy is 99.92% that is incredibly high; although the false negative rate is 1.53%. The result implies that for every 200 user sessions, more or less three intrusion attacks can infiltrate the device. Catarinucci et al. (2015) proposed a smart and sensible hospital system consisting of a hybrid-sensing network exploitation restricted application protocol, IoT sensible entryway, and a computer program to produce third parties with the power to empower health watching system patients in an endeavor to scale back the safety vulnerability of RFID in healthcare IoT infrastructure. However, data collected via IoT devices and stored in central database is very much vulnerable to be forged. This could be resolved by implementing decentralized ledger technique like blockchain, as in blockchain data blocks are recreated to distributed network nodes for the purpose of increased transparency. Quite similar to the above study, Robereto Saia proposed a unique web resolution for entities combining mobile and IoT networks into key components: entities like user devices and trackers that enable the transfer of information to the blockchain. The proposed design may be a mixture of wireless and blockchain networks that may be used for healthcare services; however, the correct implementation of such an oversized and complicated network might unlock potential constraints; as an example, it is going to be tough to minimize blockchain procedure overhead (Saia et al., 2019). Esposito et al. (2018) in their study explored healthcare data privacy and security through the introduction of various types of data structure in blockchain technology. Although, because of overhead issue of storing immense healthcare data within the blockchain, the study uses marginal data for transaction. However, data protection cannot be granted by this alone. Reducing the overhead of blockchain technology execution in small-area health networks may be a tough prospect since it desires huge computing resources to include blocks within the chain following through cryptographic logical mining algorithms like Proof-of-Work, which requires enormous computational effort. Dorri et al. (2016) came up with a unique lightweight design for networks, comprising of multiple IoT devices to beat such a haul. In this unique design for network, a local computer device is utilized as a miner, and several IoT devices conglomerate with each other in a way that one is designated as cluster head to limit access verification using policy header. This design enables the policy header to maintain upgraded access control record which is further regulated by network operator. Moreover, this research utilized a shared overspread network wherein several data owners are allowed to insert information or data into the blocks which are administered by one administrator. However, this may result in a lack of reliability among users. The review paper of Khan and Salah (2018) recognized various privacy and security threats in the present IoT environment for further research, including protection while upgrading software of billions of IoT devices for example healthcare, where blockchain technology can be utilized to increase safety and security of data. Protection and safety of very important IoT infrastructure and confidential information can mitigate attainable security and privacy issues; for instance, in mid-2016, details like master card numbers, personal information, and social insurance number of around 3.62 million patients were compromised in Banner Health, Arizona. The above example infers that primitive security systems offer protection; however, complete tamper-proof systems are difficult to attain. Among different progressive innovations, blockchain technology is contemplated by numerous people as an attainable resolution to be applied in medium and small-scale IoT systems[5] in healthcare.

4.4.5.2 Blockchain Use Cases in the Internet of Medical Things Lack of Standardization

The adoption of state-of-art IoMT technology by the healthcare industry is rapidly accelerating. Apart from the on-prem medical equipment of the healthcare provider, remote data capturing through IoMT devices enable patient condition monitoring and

---

[5] Top 10 Biggest Healthcare Data Breaches of All Time. Available online: https://www.healthcareitnews.com/news/3-phishing-hacks-breach-20000-catawba-valley-patient-records.

prescribing further curative actions. This has become a building block for telehealth surveillance applications as biosignals can be captured through internet-enabled medical devices (Pirbhulal et al., 2018). Hence secure transmission of medical data is essential. This problem stems from the fact that communication protocol and platforms are not standardized, and IoMT device manufacturers are still following their self-developed data transmission methods and tools. Hence this heterogeny has limited secure data transmission in the current state of affairs. Blockchain methodology can be used to limit the unauthorized access to data transmission over open or third-party network as communication protocol doesn't degrade the blockchain efficacy. It would require a huge computational exercise and access to more than 50% of computing nodes consent to edit even a single data block across the whole blockchain network.[6]

4.5 CONCLUSION

Blockchain technology is becoming famous day by day and succeeded in attracting the attention of not only individuals but also organizations for all kinds of activities. Blockchain is very much effective in metamorphosing the traditional industry, which incorporates auditability, decentralization, inconspicuousness, and perseverance (Gatteschi et al., 2018). Recent medical realities and challenges have brought roadblocks of the healthcare sector to limelight: fake drugs, disorganized logistics, inefficacious and unsecured data management and sharing, challenge of data privacy, etc. Unfortunately, data management systems in healthcare sector slow down the speed of imparting treatments, public resentment, and substandard health management. These inefficiencies can be worked out by inflating potentiality of the data management with the use of blockchain technology. Moreover, blockchain technology can keep information with respect to the origin of the product and can share with the related stakeholders in a transparent manner (Mattke et al., 2019).

Furthermore, blockchain technology can be utilized across various operations in healthcare sector; for example, clinical trials, EHR medical, genomics medicine, vaccine supply, and tracking along with IoT which can facilitate superior tracking in the pharma sector (Jayaraman et al., 2019). Blockchain enhances better tracking of vaccines and medicines; facilitates superior data collection,, storage, and exhortation; and allows lucidity in the exchange of several medical information and data in the process of medical trials and better medicine recalls (Mackey & Nayyar, 2017). This chapter is a sincere attempt to explore some of the major challenges and complexities with respect to medical supply chain; furthermore, an attempt is also been made to explore several available blockchain technologies, and how they are competent enough to come up with some applicable solutions to supply chain in health sector. For instance, spurious drug is a crucial challenge around the world.

Pharma co-surveillance blockchain systems are developed, which are capable of revolutionizing the complete logistics in the pharma sector. Hyperledger fabric platform which works on blockchain facilitates proper supply chain and drug records (Jamil et al., 2019). Gcoin blockchain system addresses double-spending and

---

[6] Internet of Medical Things (IoMT): The Future of Healthcare. Available online: https://igniteoutsourcing.com/healthcare/internet-of-medical-things-iomt-examples/.

counterfeiting. This blockchain system is entirely based on consensus nodes without the presence of any central regulatory body (Tseng et al., 2018). On the same note, blockchain technology is competent enough in the construct of a vaccine tracking blockchain, which could build trust and transparency among various stakeholders (Yong et al., 2019). A healthcare blockchain system facilitates the distribution of the data covering all nodes but restricts its visibility via encrypted keys among limited stakeholders (Sylim et al., 2018).

Techniques based on blockchain enhance data credibility and integrity, along with the access and exchange of health records and management of medical data in the biomedical domain (Drosatos & Kaldoudi, 2019). Tracing systems in use, like barcodes and RFID, are not competent enough to curtail the problem of tampering, as these systems send codes as fixed values which are not tamper proof and can be edited by counterfeiters. Another health care component which also requires immediate attention is medical claims and billing, and can be tackled by providing systems aiding transparency. Blockchain improves the credibility of findings from clinical trials, which are often compromised due to restricted and substandard publication and missing data. Blockchain technology is very much capable of reshaping the entire healthcare sector. It will not only bring transparency in various health care processes but will also enhance the quality of healthcare services.

REFERENCES

Alhadhrami, Z.; Alghfeli, S.; Alghfeli, M.; Abedlla, J.A.; Shuaib, K. Introducing blockchains for healthcare. *In Proceedings of the 2017 International Conference on Electrical and Computing Technologies and Applications (ICECTA)*, Ras Al Khaimah, UAE, 19–21 November 2017; pp. 1–4.

Aloqaily, M.; Otoum, S.; Al Ridhawi, I.; Jararweh, Y. An intrusion detection system for connected vehicles in smart cities. *Ad Hoc Netw.* 2019, 90, 101842.

Benchoufi, M.; Ravaud, P. Blockchain technology for improving clinical research quality. *Trials* 2017, 18, 335.

Benchoufi, M.; Porcher, R.; Ravaud, P. Blockchain protocols in clinical trials: Transparency and traceability of consent. *F1000Research* 2017, 6, 66.

Bocek, T.; Rodrigues, B.B.; Strasser, T.; Stiller, B. Blockchains everywhere: A use-case of blockchains in the pharma supply-chain. *In Proceedings of the 2017 IFIP/IEEE Symposium on Integrated Network and Service Management (IM)*, Lisbon, Portugal, 8–12 May 2017, pp. 772–777.

Catarinucci, L.; De Donno, D.; Mainetti, L.; Palano, L.; Patrono, L.; Stefanizzi, M.L.; Tarricone, L. An IoT-aware architecture for smart healthcare systems. *IEEE Internet Things J.* 2015, 2, 515–526.

Chang, S.E.; Chen, Y.C.; Lu, M.F. Supply chain reengineering using blockchain technology: A case of smart contract based tracking process. *Technol. Forecasting Social Change* 2019, 144, 1–11.

Chiuchisan, I.; Costin, H.N.; Geman, O. Adopting the internet of things technologies in health care systems. *In Proceedings of the 2014 International Conference and Exposition on Electrical and Power Engineering (EPE)*, Iasi, Romania, 16–18 October 2014, pp. 532–535.

Choi, T.M. Supply chain financing using blockchain: Impacts on supply chains selling fashionable products. *Ann. Oper. Res.* 2020, (in press). doi: 10.1007/s10479-020-03615-7.

Choudhury, O.; Fairoza, N.; Sylla, I.; Das, A. A blockchain framework for managing and monitoring data in multi-site clinical trials. arXiv 2019, arXiv:1902.03975.

De Vries, J. The shaping of inventory systems in health services: A stakeholder analysis. *Int. J. Prod. Econ.* 2011, 133(1), 60–69.

Deisingh, A.K. Pharmaceutical counterfeiting. *Analyst* 2005, 130, 271–279.

Dimitrov, D.V. Medical internet of things and big data in healthcare. *Healthc. Inform. Res.* 2016, 22, 156–163.

Dorri, A.; Kanhere, S.S.; Jurdak, R. Blockchain in internet of things: Challenges and solutions. arXiv 2016, arXiv:1608.05187.159.

Drosatos, G.; Kaldoudi, E. Blockchain applications in the biomedical domain: A scoping review. *Comput. Struct. Biotechnol. J.* 2019, 17, 229–240.

Dujak, D.; Sajter, D. Blockchain applications in supply chain. In Kawa, A.; Maryniak, A. (Eds.), *SMART Supply Network*, pp. 21–46. Springer: Cham, Switzerland, 2019.

Esposito, C.; De Santis, A.; Tortora, G.; Chang, H.; Choo, K.K.R. Blockchain: A panacea for healthcare cloud-based data security and privacy? *IEEE Cloud Comput.* 2018, 5, 31–37.

Ford, E.W.; Scanlon, D. P. Promise and problems with supply chain management approaches to health care purchasing. *Acad. Manage. Proc. No.* 2006, 1, A1–A6.

Funk, E.; Riddell, J.; Ankel, F.; Cabrera, D. Blockchain technology: A data framework to improve validity, trust, and accountability of information exchange in health professions education. *Acad. Med.* 2018, 93, 1791–1794.

Gaggioli, A. Blockchain technology: Living in a decentralized everything. *Cyberpsychol. Behav. Soc. Netw.* 2018, 21, 65–66.

Gatteschi, V.; Lamberti, F.; Demartini, C.; Pranteda, C.; Santamaría, V. Blockchain and smart contracts for insurance: Is the technology mature enough? *Future Internet* 2018, 10, 20.

Griggs, K.N.; Ossipova, O.; Kohlios, C.P.; Baccarini, A.N.; Howson, E.A.; Hayajneh, T. Healthcare blockchain system using smart contracts for secure automated remote patient monitoring. *J. Med. Syst.* 2018, 42, 130.

Haghi, M.; Thurow, K.; Stoll, R. Wearable devices in medical internet of things: Scientific research and commercially available devices. *Healthc. Inform. Res.* 2017, 23, 4–15.

Hölbl, M.; Kompara, M.; Kamišalić, A.; Zlatolas, L.N. A systematic review of the use of blockchain in healthcare. *Symmetry* 2018, 10, 470.

Ichikawa, D.; Kashiyama, M.; Ueno, T. Tamper-resistant mobile health using blockchain technology. *JMIR mHealth uHealth* 2017, 5, e111.

Idrees, S.M.; Nowostawski, M.; Jameel, R. Blockchain-based digital contact tracing apps for COVID-19 pandemic management: Issues, challenges, solutions, and future directions. *JMIR Med. Inf.,* 2021, 9(2), e25245.

Isojarvi, J.; Wood, H.; Lefebvre, C.; Glanville, J. Challenges of identifying unpublished data from clinical trials: Getting the best out of clinical trials registers and other novel sources. *Res. Synth. Methods* 2018, 9, 561–578.

Jamil, F.; Hang, L.; Kim, K.; Kim, D. A novel medical blockchain model for drug supply chain integrity management in a smart hospital. *Electronics.* 2019, 8(5), 505.

Jayaraman, R.; AlHammadi, F.; Simsekler, M.C.E. Managing product recalls in healthcare supply chain. *In Proceedings of the 2018 IEEE International Conference on Industrial Engineering and Engineering Management (IEEM)*, Bangkok, Thailand, 16–19 December 2018, pp. 293–297.

Jayaraman, R.; Saleh, K.; King, N. Improving opportunities in healthcare supply chain processes via the internet of things and blockchain technology. *Int. J. Healthcare Informat. Syst. Informat. (IJHISI)* 2019, 14(2), 49–65.

Jo, B.; Khan, R.; Lee, Y.S. Hybrid blockchain and internet-of-things network for underground structure health monitoring. *Sensors* 2018, 18, 4268.

Khan, M.A.; Salah, K. IoT security: Review, blockchain solutions, and open challenges. *Future Gen. Comput. Syst.* 2018, 82, 395–411.

Kim, C.; Kim, H.J. A study on healthcare supply chain management efficiency: Using bootstrap data envelopment analysis. *Health Care Manage. Sci.* 2019, 22(3), 1–15.

Kshetri, N. Blockchain's roles in strengthening cybersecurity and protecting privacy. *Telecommun. Policy*, 41(10), 1027–1038, 2017. doi: 10.1016/j.telpol.2017.09.003.

Kumar, R.; Agarwal, A.; Shubhankar, B. Counterfeit drug detection: Recent strategies and analytical perspectives. *Int. J. Pharma Res. Health Sci.* 2018, 6, 2351–2358.

Landry, S.; Beaulieu, M. The challenges of hospital supply chain management, from central stores to nursing units. In Denton, B. T. (Ed.), *Handbook of Healthcare Operations Management*, pp. 465–482. Springer New York, 2013.

Landry, S.; Philippe, R. How logistics can service healthcare. *Supply Chain Forum Int. J.* 2004, 5(2), 24–30.

Lee, S.M.; Lee, D.; Schniederjans, M.J. Supply chain innovation and organizational performance in the healthcare industry. *Int. J. Oper. Prod. Manage.* 2011, 31, 1193–1214.

Lin, I.C.; Liao, T.C. A survey of blockchain security issues and challenges. *IJ Netw. Secur.* 2017, 19, 653–659.

Mackey, T.K.; Nayyar, G. A review of existing and emerging digital technologies to combat the global trade in fake medicines. *Expert Opin. Drug Saf.* 2017, 16(5), 587–602.

Macrinici, D.; Cartofeanu, C.; Gao, S. Smart contract applications within blockchain technology: A systematic mapping study. *Telemat. Inform.* 2018, 35, 2337–2354.

Marucheck, A.; Greis, N.; Mena, C.; Cai, L. Product safety and security in the global supply chain: Issues, challenges and research opportunities. *J. Oper. Manage.* 2011, 29, 707–720.

Mattke, J.; Hund, A.; Maier, C.; Weitzel, T. How an enterprise blockchain application in the US pharmaceuticals supply chain is saving lives. *MIS Quart. Executive.* 2019, 18(4), 246–261.

McKone-Sweet, K.E.; Hamilton, P.; Willis, S.B. The ailing healthcare supply chain: A prescription for change. *J. Supply Chain Manage.* 2005, 41(1), 4–17.

Michael, J.; Cohn, A.; Butcher, J.R. Blockchain technology. 2018. Available online: https://www.steptoe.com/images/content/1/7/v3/171269/LIT-FebMar18-Feature-Blockchain.pdf (accessed on 20 March 2019).

Montecchi, M.; Plangger, K.; Etter, M. It's real, trust me! Establishing supply chain provenance using blockchain. *Bus. Horiz.* 2019, 62(3), 283–293.

Moosavi, S.R.; Gia, T.N.; Rahmani, A.M.; Nigussie, E.; Virtanen, S.; Isoaho, J.; Tenhunen, H. SEA: A secure and efficient authentication and authorization architecture for IoT-based healthcare using smart gateways. *Procedia Comput. Sci.* 2015, 52, 452–459.

Narayanaswami, C.; Nooyi, R.; Raghavan, S.G.; Viswanathan, R. Blockchain anchored supply chain automation. *IBM J. Res. Dev.* 2019, 63, 7.1–7.11.

Nausheen, F.; Begum, S.H. Healthcare IoT: Benefits, vulnerabilities and solutions. *In Proceedings of the 2018 IEEE 2nd International Conference on Inventive Systems and Control (ICISC)*, Coimbatore, India, 19–20 January 2018, pp. 517–522.

Nikoloudakis, Y.; Pallis, E.; Mastorakis, G.; Mavromoustakis, C.X.; Skianis, C.; Markakis, E.K. Vulnerability assessment as a service for fog-centric ICT ecosystems: A healthcare use case. *Peer-to-Peer Netw. Appl.* 2019; vol. 5, 1–9.

Nugent, T.; Upton, D.; Cimpoesu, M. Improving data transparency in clinical trials using blockchain smart contracts. *F1000Research* 2016, 5, 2541.

Pilkington, M. 11 Blockchain technology: Principles and applications. In Olleros, F.X.; Zhegu, M. (Eds), *Research Handbook on Digital Transformations*, p. 225. Edward Elgar: Cheltenham, UK, 2016.

Pirbhulal, S.; Wu, W.; Li, G. A biometric security model for wearable healthcare. *In Proceedings of the 2018 IEEE International Conference on Data Mining Workshops (ICDMW)*, Singapore, 17–20 November 2018; pp. 136–143.

Plotnikov, V.; Kuznetsova, V. The prospects for the use of digital technology "blockchain" in the pharmaceutical market. *In MATEC Web of Conferences; EDP Sciences*, Ho Chi Minh, Vietnam, 2018; vol. 193, p. 02029.

Privett, N.; Gonsalvez, D. The top ten global health supply chain issues: Perspectives from the field. *Oper. Res. Health Care* 2014, 3(4), 226–230.

Qiao, R.; Zhu, S.; Wang, Q.; Qin, J. Optimization of dynamic data traceability mechanism in internet of things based on consortium blockchain. *Int. J. Distrib. Sensor Networks*, 2018, 14(12), 1550147718819072.

Rahman, M.A.; Hassanain, E.; Rashid, M.M.; Barnes, S.J.; Hossain, M.S. Spatial blockchain-based secure mass screening framework for children with dyslexia. *IEEE Access* 2018, 6, 61876–61885.

Saia, R.; Carta, S.; Recupero, D.; Fenu, G. Internet of Entities (IoE): A blockchain-based distributed paradigm for data exchange between wireless-based devices. *In Proceedings of the 8th International Conference on Sensor Networks (SENSORNETS 2019)*, Prague, Cxech Republic, 26–27 January 2019.

Scalise, D. Building an efficient supply chain. *Hosp. Health Networks*, 2005, 79(8), 47–52.

Schöner, M.M.; Kourouklis, D.; Sandner, P.; Gonzalez, E.; Förster, J. *Blockchain Technology in the Pharmaceutical Industry*. Frankfurt School Blockchain Center: Frankfurt, Germany, 2017.

Shae, Z.; Tsai, J.J. On the design of a blockchain platform for clinical trial and precision medicine. *In Proceedings of the 2017 IEEE 37th International Conference on Distributed Computing Systems (ICDCS)*, Atlanta, GA, 5–8 June 2017, pp. 1972–1980.

Sylim, P.; Liu, F.; Marcelo, A.; Fontelo, P. Blockchain technology for detecting falsified and substandard drugs in distribution: Pharmaceutical supply chain intervention. *J. Med. Internet Res.* 2018, 7(9), e10163.

Toyoda, K.; Mathiopoulos, P.T.; Sasase, I.; Ohtsuki, T. A novel blockchain-based product ownership management system (POMS) for anti-counterfeits in the post supply chain. *IEEE Access* 2017, 5, 17465–17477.

Tseng, J.-H.; Liao, Y.-C.; Chong, B.; Liao, S.-W. Governance on the drug supply chain via Gcoin blockchain. *Int. J. Environ. Res. Public Health*. 2018, 15(6), 1055.

Westerkamp, M.; Victor, F.; Kupper, A. Tracing manufacturing processes using blockchain-based token compositions. *Dig. Commun. Netw.* 2019, 6(2), 167–176.

World Health Organisation. WHO Global Surveillance and Monitoring System for Substandard and Falsified Medical Products; World Health Organisation: Geneva, Switzerland, 2017.

Yang, R.; Yu, F.R.; Si, P.; Yang, Z.; Zhang, Y. Integrated blockchain and edge computing systems: A survey, some research issues and challenges. *IEEE Commun. Surv. Tutor.* 2019, 21, 1508–1532.

Yong, B.; Shen, J.; Liu, X.; Li, F.; Chen, H.; Zhou, Q. An intelligent blockchain-based system for safe vaccine supply and supervision. *Int. J. Inf. Manage.* 2019, 52, 102024.

Zhang, J.; Xue, N.; Huang, X. A secure system for pervasive social network-based healthcare. *IEEE Access* 2016, 4, 9239–9250.

Zhu, Q.; Kouhizadeh, M. Blockchain technology, supply chain information, and strategic product deletion management. *IEEE Eng. Manage. Rev.* 2019, 47, 36–44.

5 Digital Transformation in Healthcare: Innovation and Technologies

Suruchi Singh, Pankaj Bhatt,
Satish Kumar Sharma, and S. Rabiu
Glocal University

CONTENTS

DOI: 10.1201/9781003141471-5

5.1   INTRODUCTION

Digital transformation (DT) mentions a procedure that will help promote the system by facilitating the beneficial alteration of its possession by combining particular computing and linkage technologies (Vial, 2019). DT is the other in the field of health management, when a person starts to take advantage of the forte.. It is the procedure of bringing up digital technologies to the whole health management commerce-remunerator performance supplier and member associated. Additionally, cultural modification and empower development in commerce cleverness, as a result, developed performance quality, victim adventure, and expense deduction (HCL Technology Q&A, n.d.). DM in health care is a useful collision of technology in health management. The digital transformation in Healthcare (HC) initiates additional trade chances and produces another modern trade prototype to communicate matter in medical conversation benefit generation and more issues associated with, within the other, the older community (Elton & O'Riordan, 2016). The US health management market is enormous and there its digital clinical market is anticipated to get to 504.4 billion USD in 2025 from 86.4 billion at a Compound annual growth rate (CARG) of 29.26%; nevertheless, the demand and the entire photograph of recent digital health management scenery changes the level of exercise in the year of 2020 (Jayaraman et al., 2020). In modern methodical literature review, again Digital Transformation (DT)in healthcare displays how investigation on this subject matters up sewing for the fast 20 years ago and draws attention to the almost all standard technology-associated analysis object with this kingdom. India's health management market is among the rapid developing spot, a profuse develop almost 25% in current years and correctly so. The market standard of medical technology is attached at million and anticipated to table of ones under 50% of the time by 2020 the disturbance in the region is handled by technology revolution together with IT, biomedical analysis, health management transport prototype of health management people and education supplier and anticipation for a more to the epidemiological spread (HCL Technology Q&A, n.d.).

5.2 WHY DIGITAL TRANSFORMATION FOR HEALTH CARE

By tremendous volume of victims attending all help facilities, it is tough for those organizations to attract digital procedures and resolutions to supplier complete and rapid victims. More especially interacting with an enormous volume of victims' details and history (Hakuna matata tech, 2020). It is used to alter frequently (operate manually) almost medical-based health industries influenced the victims' management. The industries all participate with seasoned DT services invest in digital resolution to supply rapid and effective services to the victims. Firstly, digital technologies currently anticipated to promote the standard of management and performance competence rigid quick medical and monitoring assignment joint to the judgment transportation judgment and exactness of medical cure. The acceptance of technological revolution such as easily wearable equipment enjoy health apps has mostly collided with multinational exercise and locates a victim in the Health Management (HM) system. These and some other solutions hold promotion in huge details and details' investigation leading to more than the probability of privatized management. Second, four significant resemblances interrelate amongst victims and customers to show the traditional caretakers of the HM market. HM supplier legislators, in collaboration with third-party DT generators, could not change procedure in the midst of these traditional organizations on their own, but rather update all HM regions. (Friedrichsen & Mühl-Benninghaus, 2013). Different current market participants disrupted the quality sequence of telemedicine commerce: telecoms organizations and mobile entrepreneurs, pharmaceutical industries and medication manufacturers, and equipment and policy handling sorts (Wright & Androuchko, 1996; FPFIS team, 2013).

5.3 DIGITAL TRANSFORMATION TECHNOLOGIES IN HEALTH CARE

1. Artificial intelligence
2. Augmented reality and virtual reality
3. Cloud computing
4. Blockchain technology
5. IoT
6. Telemedicine
7. Robotics
8. Chatbots
9. Alexa
10. Big data (HCL Technology Q&A, n.d.)

5.3.1 ARTIFICIAL INTELLIGENCE

The life of an artificial intelligence doctor is made so much simpler. Victims and clinic executives interrelate hereditary codes to the help of the robotic in the treatment identifying the chronic disease and regulating risk judgement by executing chores that are generally performed by humanity at a low cost and in a short period of time after seeking a connection. AI is a renovate and re-energize recent health management via a modern device that can understand forecast, pickup, and proceed (Takyar, 2020). AI supplies a figure of values better than medical resolution makers and customary logic; investigation procedure more perfect and error-free by the time they interconnected with coaching details. It can permit humankind to obtain extraordinary perception to the custody procedure surgery changeable victims' result and medical checkup. AI is better than a DM direction in health management. For the therapeutic resolution synopsis, AI acts, and industrial actors do not wait to spend millions in it. It is expected that the health management AI energizing types of equipment market will reach USD 34 billion by 2025, indicating that this technology will shape almost all facets of the industry.

For nearly all victims, AI in medicine evokes a memory of Japanese nurse robots. However, today, various American versions also search, Moxi, a helpful clinic droid created by daily duty like Tekken to assist human nurses. Providing genuine AI ability better analyzed in the district, such as exactness drugs medical diagnostics, drugs found, and genomics, such as cancerous victims used to collect unimaginative surgery and more nonfulfillment rates. Currently grateful to AI globally, acknowledging those having opportunities to privatize treatment customize heredity makeup and opinions on what AI power computer scheme does for oncology. It examines thousands of pathology images of different cancers to supply great precise medical checkup and a forecast the likely anticancer medicines, and in clinical imaging diagnostics, technology-assisted radiographers mark data that get away from humankind's eye.

Additionally, topmost pharmaceutical and biotechnology industries are employing device coaching method to reduce the medicine evolution round. Present discovery displays that AI can slash initial medicines finding duration by 4 years against the companies' median and reduce the expenses of about 60%. Overall, AI is expected to generate USD 150 billion per annum to save health management by 2026; startups are jumping on this opportunity earlier; since 2000, India's figure of energetic AI startups has increased about 14 times (Reddy, 2020).

Here Are Some Methods of AI to Bring Health Management Modification

- **Medical Checkup and Deducting Inaccuracy**

  Around 10% of deaths in the United States of America are a result of clinical mistakes and inaccuracies in illness diagnosis. AI is the most astonishing electrified technologies promised to improve the trusted healthcare system and decrease many faults. Massive caseloads and incomplete clinical data may be a factor in human mortality mistake. Nevertheless, AI can assist forecast and investigate illness rapidly more than any other medical professionals, such as one-off investigation of an AI prototype employed procedure and profound acquirement to investigate cancerous breast disease at a higher rate than 11 pathologists. Breast cancer is discovered to be second significant causes of cancer in females in USA, and screening mammography has discovered to deduct the numbers of morality, computer-assisted detection, and medical checkup software constructed in the 1990s Ashish radiographer advanced the forecasting of data analysis of screening mammography.

Unfortunately, details proposed that initial CAD program could not bring development in functioning. Nonetheless, the great success of deep acquisition in viewable material observation acknowledgement profound acquisition equipment aided radiographers in pushing mammography screening.

- **Analytics for Pathology Images**

  Vital means of medical checkup are supplied by pathologist suppliers all over the spread parturition management. Seventy percentage of all health management conclusions based on pathology outcomes. Some other places in between 70% and 75% of all figures in an HER come from pathology outcomes the correct we obtain, and we will gain accurate analysis. We will become the finest; a single digital pathology fallacy must accompany virtual pathology and AI opportunities. Proscia uses artificial intelligence to find the models in cancer cells. It allows pathologists to remove congestion from the management of statistics and supports Ai-empower resemblance analysis to connect the end of statistics, which would improve cancer investigation and treatment and AI and facilitates binary search character of efficiency in slides before examining the details by doctors.

- **Converting mobile selfies into efficient tools for diagnosis**

  Controlling the ability of transportable tools, the specialists presume that taking a picture with a cell phone and other roots can be vital accessories to clinical standard medical imagine more especially in promoting the counties since the standard of cell phones is getting development. Annually mobile phone can supply a picture which is qualified to investigate via AI procedure. Some investigators of UK half-constructed devices that can be able to identify the developmental illness through investigation pictures of the children's faces. The procedure can be able to organize individual peculiarity, for instance, the eyes and nose of the children's arrangement jawline and other ones ascribed that showing congenital disabilities of abnormality of craniofacial. Consequently, It is an outstanding opportunity for us to turn a variety of figures to a treasures understanding cell phones can be employed together pictures of the skin lesions, wound, medications, infections, or eyes to assist inadequately service places to control a scarcity of expertise while deducting the period to analysis for other criticism.

- **Management of Electronic Health Records**

  The figure (made of victim information, current investigation findings, and medical checkup data) is referred to as an electronic health record (EHR), and it is constantly developed in large quantities in health management facilities. Artificial intelligence in HERs assists syndicates in gaining understanding in order to collaborate with sufferers and announce conclusion. When combined with AI, an electronic clinical record platform may provide health management employees with the capacity to direct their analysis rather of relying on the inclusion of figures. Manually in HERs, AI enables health management personnel to detect current figures and also to extract valuable knowledge that can be used to provide advice. AI in health management personnel enables details in EHRs to be converted to nearly enough assistance that can benefit health management personnel using AI-energized EHRs. For instance, if pharmaceuticals really aren't healthy for patients based on extrapolating of victim genes, the AI-based programme may have alternative suitable hiding.

- **Production of Medications and Vaccine**

    Let us comprehend the round of medicine buildout before knowing how AI technology helped buildout medicine industry gate was determined a target protein responsible for illness caused? They inspect that protein consciousness for an extended period if not there is the possibility of missing a considerable amount of money on incorrect protein and then investigate protein make an effort to search. A molecule or a compound will damage the compound itself. Proteins should be comfortable to turn differently in order to uncover the cause of disease protein effectively. In the procedure, the fruitless compound is tossed away and only guarded, and well-organized compounds prosper for the improvement of medicine the whole procedure of manual period consuming; hence, AI appears into the image. There are hundreds and thousands of molecules, and humanity analyst cannot examine the molecules manually, even now in the absence of examining every molecule is impossible to detect which of the molecule to suit for the main application to use for the treatment of such particular illness. To hire AI experts, the framework must be fed first. After that, any other Automation system will continually learn skills from starting figures and find another substance mostly used to combat disease. Likewise, the vaccine can be promoted and analyzed effectively by taking advantage of artificial intelligence.

- **Repetitive Workflow Automation**

    The technology of AI is guaranteed to convert the current function of the health management organization managing surrounding. Unstrained to duty on high-rank individuals from qualifying investigates to details transferred and nonjudicial stamp, all the things can be automatic; consequently, employees can highlight providing best services to victims. Olive may be integrated into a present clinic software, either of the AI as support equipment, withdrawing the need for expensive idle time or mixture.

- **Notifying Physicians When Patient Victims in Trouble**

    Various clinics globally employing Google's in-depth mind health AI to help operate victims from medical checkup to therapy expertly. The deep mind health system informs physicians by the time victims' health aggravated and can even help in medical checkup of illness investigation by an enormous set of figures related signs. By assembling victims' symptoms and recording them into the in-depth mind program, the physician can determine the illness very expertly and rapidly (HCL Technology Q&A, n.d.).

5.3.2 DIGITAL REALITY AND AUGMENTED REALITY (AR)

The employees of health management were in haste to recognize the value of AR technologies. Knowledge was the explicit request of augmented reality in the health management area. Health management employees should acquire a large sum of knowledge of human anatomy and physiology. The AR technology offers the trainee the chances to see and interrelate the three-dimensional rendition of bodies. Nevertheless, health management employees alone commented reality-aided and assured immense benefit as a device for the knowledge of victims permit health personal to assist victims in comprehending the treatment method and how drugs act latter-day physicians employ different technologies to see the side where they work on. However, instead, augmented reality can plan a three-dimensional rendition of the victim's anatomy to the area of surgeons' prospects. It seems to improve the accuracy and outcome for patients. A non-theoretical demand of virtual reality veins is in sighting several patients are really no discomfort with blood infusions. The acquaintance is substantially more inadequate when vein could not be located from the victims need to "inserted" several times. (TD_Madison, 2020).

ACC Vein, for example, now has a Sic-kbay employee who can create a map of a victim's vein up to their epidermis, making it very easy for health management personnel to get the vein immediately. (Apple Inc, n.d.). Cable Labs, a high-speed internet company investigation group, are at the most critical investigation to the request of augmented reality their sights in the upcoming AR in health Management management the closest upcoming time the best region supplies engrossing perception to the method enhances in network technology. Reality will alter the standard of life for elders. Other ones rely on health management organization. Even though augmented reality is employed daily by the health personnel employees all over the USA, there is a method to go to previous to the enormous chances for commerce that comprehends augmented reality and having an insight initiate introducing modern AR products and request (Apple Inc, n.d.).

The virtual reality is a technology that employs the computer created an imitation of a three-dimensional picture or a setting which can permit a human being to listen. Insights interrelate via employing the specific device for instance headsets (Microsoft HoloLens, n.d.).

The techniques create an imitated place whereby benefits can submerge in. Not like custody benefiters affiliates, Virtual reality (VR) is carrying benefits into the virtual acquaintance, a substitute of showing a curtain alone.

The health Management management organization embraces practical reality to bring the best treatment to the victims; for instance, one of the victims has been on drugs treatment weekly for almost 6 months for a duration course of cure.

During infusion, she needs to go to beach to take rest woefully and cannot go in life as is lived in reality due to her skin that was very sensitized to sunlight. Nevertheless, rather virtual reality make her to fulfill her ambition through imitating the beach-like place where she can feel massive. She sat down on the sand and can also be entertained by the sunbath. She was not the only person attracted to utilize virtual reality in the field of health management but rather many victims are in need of such acquaintance when they undergo surgery from the hospital first aid rooms. The virtual reality is blown up an anticipation to expand in the future continuously based on an investigation by GlobeNewswire. The commerce center of virtual reality in health management would get up to 7 billion USD in the year of 2026 (The Medical Futurist, 2017). Health management technology till date is in prompt stage; henceforth, the organization of health management has begun to determine where it can be employed and the challenges produced by the VR

Here's how the healthcare sector will benefit from VR: pain relief

Children's National Hospital, Washington DC, conducted a test program of pain reduction for the children who were undergoing stitches removal, sutures, and children who needed foreign body removal in emergency rooms. The program included the use of virtual reality headsets. The number of children who were tested amounted to 40, and the age group was between 7 and 23. The children were given a VR headset covered in protective gear so that the gems could be cut down. Virtual reality headset was given to each child.

After this, all the children were asked to select a scenario they prepared, and the scenarios included talking to a familiar snake and enjoying a roller coaster trip across a forest. All the VR headphones were added to the screens by the children so that parents could see everything going on. The parents were overjoyed to see that their children did not experience any pain during the whole activity. They were thrilled seeing that this VR headset could reduce the pain that their children would feel while undergoing stitches removal and foreign body removal in emergency rooms. Many health institutes have started using this VR technology for pain reduction theories because it has proved to be a persuasive technology.

- **Physical Exercise Rehab Pacing up**

    The VR technology can also be used in physical therapy. It can produce an environment that will make the patient enjoy the physical therapy, and it does this by providing an environment that is pretending or imitating an environment required for the patient to feel good during the therapy. Researchers showed that children the cerebral palsy had positive results after using VR Technology. The children improved in their ability to walk and in their body movements. Gamified approach to physical therapy has been introduced by augmented reality physical therapy's top creators, Neuro Rehab VR. The approach that has been done by the providers includes some exercises that involve a machine learning how to customize some exercises to meet the patient's therapeutic requirement. These machines are meant to make sure that each makes each exercise to meet the patient's needs of therapeutic requirements. The goal of all this is to pace up the recovery of patient occupational therapy.

- **VR models to understand challenges from the viewpoint of someone else**

    Virtual reality can be used experiencing life from the viewpoint of someone else. It enables one to realize how someone feels and help those who deal with patients to understand how they feel and how they affect the patient. It is also used by the students doing some research to understand how the disease is affecting the patient. This virtual reality stimulation is done using a VR headset and engaging with images at 360°.

This encourages one to view life from the viewpoint of someone else. The company's first labs conducted research, with the goal of transforming all users into Alfred, a 74-year-old African American suffering from high-frequency hearing impairment and molecular deterioration. When the student put on the headsets, they realized they were about in embodying Alfred even though they could make their introductions. The key was for them to say "there is something broken I cannot see, as a turn up the volume I cannot hear." This happened, and they realized they truly afraid when they said that kind of things because only Alfred could say these things to his condition therefore by using VR are imported leaves can control what we cannot see this we are stimulation now have to understand the feeling inexperience of someone suffering from a deadly disease. This occurred, and they recognized that they were indeed incarnating Alfred when they spoke these things since only Alfred could have uttered such things given his situation. Therefore, by using VR, embodied labs can control what we cannot see, what we cannot hear, and what we can see or hear. This stimulation now helps people understand the feeling and the experience of someone suffering from a deadly disease (Gordon & Catalini, 2018).

It is something that would have amazed the people 10 years ago, telling them that the use of video games could reduce pain. Now, it has been shown that the video can do real good to reduce pain. The use of virtual reality digitally transformed health. Virtual reality has many applications in changing the way that the patient is now being treated. In previous years, the doctors managed the pain of the patients in so many different ways. These included doctors handling opioids such as the candy to the patient. In postoperative pain, they used some oxytocin, Vicodin, or Percocet to reduce the pain. In this way, the pain management results in the worst current drug crisis in America's history. This has led to the estimated economic cost of 78, 5 billion. Many people are still suffering from chronic pain, and the CDC's statistics have shown that about 50 million adults in the USA still had chronic pain in 2016.

Virtual reality technology has proven to be the one most efficient to these adults than the use of the drugs. This technology has more other uses than pain management; it can manage anxiety over post-traumatic stress and stroke conditions. Virtual reality technology has proved to have more applications other than these that have been mentioned above. Some of these applications include virtual reality by doctors in residents to simulate to hone their skills or plan complicated surgeries. Wears are also motivated by this virtual reality to exercise and help children deal with the world. Many pharmacy individuals are talking about the VR, and they have found that it had so many supporting points. By 2025, it has been estimated that virtual and augmented reality will reach 5.1 billion in health care. It is advisable to all companies that want to improve their company's digital marketing strategy to consider VR technology as it has proven to be a promising technology. Virtual research technology will improve customers' sense of customers and their needs and virtually help link with products and services. It can also be used in consultation between the doctors and the patient. They have proven to save much time for the doctors. The patient is now able to contact the doctors and discuss so the relevant information using the VR. This saves much time for the doctors because before the patient comes to the doctor, they already know everything needed to treat the patient. Virtual reality can be used for medical staff training and improving their skills (Reddy, 2020; Innovative Architects, n.d.).

5.3.3 CLOUD COMPUTING

Spending on the rise together with IT, the cloud-based electronic clinical data (ECD) is the origin to hold a collision on the medical organization, with all this regard and risky cloud computing modifying health management continuously in the present time.

Firstly, as a software as a service (SaaS), the cloud enables to allow health management industries on seeking service providers and supplies rapid entrance to commerce application and accomplished customer relationship care(CRC). As social amenities as service (SaaS), cloud resolution can be able to permit on-seeking computing and massive storage for clinical provision. Moreover, in platform as a service (PaaS), the cloud itself can permit security to improve region for Web-based service and improvements of Web-based applications. Modifying health and via the cloud is practically superior to just pull up clinical data from different computers at any particular time, anywhere, and on any mobile phone device. It also has the effect of enabling the ability to link clinical regions and cloud services specifically to disseminate victim's clinical figures over the worldwide system of interconnected networking. (Innovative Architects, n.d.).

Due to the elastic and virtually unlimited scalability, high availability, and accessibility of data at an affordable budget of cloud computing, it has many benefits to health care. It has been shown by the Atomic bomb casually commission (ABCC) research, the usage of cloud computing by healthcare stakeholders will reach 35 billion by 2022. The cumulative annual growth rate is double, and it is increasing at a rate of 16% over the 2017–2022 period. Usage of the cloud computing solution will make operations in health care to be cost-effective and convenient. Cloud computing is proving to be a promising one in health care.

The cloud has a complex infrastructure that may pose difficulties in understanding though it offers on-demand computing by utilizing the latest technology to cause independence of access and use networked information, applications, and resources. Most users have concluded that cloud computing is the best choice to use for their healthcare business. It is cheaper than using many computers in different rooms. These computers would need proper hardware, updated software and accessibility to the network to upload, preserve, and retrieve patients. The healthcare IT solutions have done so many things that have benefited health care. These included improvement of the security and safeguards.

Now, the cloud computing solutions, service providers, and carriers and health organization are relaxed knowing that they are protected from the potential loss of control over certain sensitive information about the patience (Innovative Architects, n.d.).

5.3.4 BLOCKCHAIN TECHNOLOGY

A blockchain is a disseminated, public record, recording exchange and following resources, and of which permanence is ensured by a shared organization of PCs, not by any brought together position. Numerous parts of blockchain innovation, for example, the unchanging nature of the information put away in a blockchain, are drawing the medical services area's consideration, and blushing possibilities for some, accessible cases are being examined. Blockchain innovation is required to improve clinical record the executives and the protection guarantee measure and quicken clinical and biomedical examination and advance biomedical and medical care information records (Kuo et al., 2017). These desires depend on blockchain innovation's critical viewpoints, for example, decentralized administration, permanent review trail, information provenance, strength, and improved security and protection. Albeit a few prospects have been examined, the most outstanding development that can be accomplished with blockchain innovation is the recuperation of information sub-jects' correct. Clinical information should be controlled, worked, and permitted by information subjects other than emergency clinics. This is a critical idea of patient-focused interoperability that varies from regular organization-driven interoperability (Gordon & Catalini, 2018).

5.3.5 INTERNET OF THINGS (IoT)

Internet of Things (IoT) has begun to affect the healthcare industry through shrewd associated gadgets, frameworks, and things that are utilized by billions of clients to use the information and help them make all the more ideal, explicit, and contextual-ized choices. IoT in the healthcare business has opened entryways for some chances. As indicated by a market conjecture, The IoT healthcare market is worth $158.07 billion, with 50 billion-associated gadgets by 2020. Utilize wearable devices to col-lect data about health, hence supporting professionals in comprehending the whole picture of the disease, and so on. (Gordon & Catalini, 2018).

IoT is changing the clinical services industry by modifying people's collaboration in giving clinical services plans. Since IoT has made coordinated efforts with experts successful and less complicated, it has improved patient satisfaction and responsibil-ity. Moreover, far-off checking of patients' prosperity helps hinder re-assertions and decrease the range of stay in the crisis facility. IoT can similarly decrease clinical services costs and improve treatment results. IoT is changing the medical services industry by rebuilding individuals' cooperation in giving medical services arrange-ments. Execution of IoT in medical services benefits doctors, clinics, patients, and insurance agencies (Yoon, 2019).

5.3.5.1 IoT for Physicians

With home-checking gear embedded with IoT sensors and wearable contraptions, spe-cialists can ceaselessly screen patients' prosperity. IoT permits medical care experts to turn out to be more vigilant and connect with patients proactively. Information accumulated from IoT gadgets can help specialists decide the best treatment measure for patients and get expected results.

5.3.5.2 IoT for Patients

Gadget, for example, wellness groups and remotely associated pulse observing sleeves give patients admittance to customized consideration. IoT gadgets are utilized to remind regular checkups, carbohydrate content, number of steps required in a day, circulatory strain, pulse, and significantly more. IoT empowers continuous distant checking and is helpful for older patients. It utilizes a ready component and sends a warning to concerned medical services suppliers and relatives.

5.3.5.3 IoT for Hospitals and Clinics

Aside from following patients' well-being, IoT gadgets can be utilized in numerous different regions in clinics. IoT gadgets installed with sensors are utilized for check-ing the constant area of clinical hardware, including nebulizers, wheelchairs, oxygen siphons, and other gears.

Clinics likewise need to manage the spread of contamination that is the essential worry for them. IoT-based cleanliness-checking gadgets help with keeping patients from getting the contamination. For instance, brilliant IoT-empowered cameras can identify if patients are washing or disinfecting their hands before taking dinner or drug or guests are not sitting near the patient. Additionally, IoT gadgets can help in overseeing resources, for instance, checking fridge temperature and moistness.

5.3.6 TELEMEDICINE

Telemedicine is a superb option for patients to conquer the distance between patient and supplier, admittance to dependable transportation, fracture of care because of holes in time boundaries among arrangements, and absence of medical services suppliers. A new overview shows that 90% had just begun creating or executing a telemedicine program (Gordon & Catalini, 2018). Telemedicine development is one of the main changes in the US medical services market. In a major nation like the USA, where admittance to medical care suppliers is restricted, telemedicine is arising thoroughly. Ninety percentage of studied medical services chiefs uncovered that associations began building or coordinating a telemedicine framework. Telehealth innovation can likewise be utilized to oversee patients at great danger and empower well-being experts to follow the patient's conditions and exercises distantly utilizing IoT-based well-being sensors and wearable gadgets. It is essential to consider that the telemedicine application or arrangement ought to follow enactment focused on areas or nation. We have assembled a telemedicine application for medical services foundations that encourage specialists to cooperate with existing and new patients and patients to speak with existing specialists using video, voice, or text talk (Yoon, 2019). Telemedicine advantages are expanded admittance to mind, improve persistent consideration quality, lessen medical care costs, improve understanding commitment/fulfillment, upgraded medical care specialist co-op fulfillment, more accommodation, stretched out admittance to trained professionals and alluding doctors.

5.3.7 ROBOTICS

Robots assist clinical faculty with performing routine errands quicker to help them center around other squeezing duties. Such robotization in medical services makes operations more secure and more affordable for patients. The excellent slack of using robots in clinical services is to perform microsurgery, which individuals find hard to manage. The utilization of robots in medical care can bring a ton of preferences for example, and they could help doctors inspect patients, transport clinical supplies, help with recovery, and give Assistance to clinical supplies pressing. Likewise, it may mechanize specific cycles (Hakuna matata tech, 2020). The possibility of robots in improving medical care is not new—as right on time as 1985, there was an arrangement to change modern robots into accuracy machines for a medical procedure and past. The appearance and improvement of the Da Vinci robot in the mid-2000s and this notorious grape medical procedure video demonstrate how far innovative advancement has come. Be that as it may, regardless of how great, advanced mechanics in medical care is a framework constrained by people. The genuine enchantment of the 21st-century robo-specialist will come from human-made consciousness frameworks that can adapt so much that it will beat the best specialists by joining all the accessible information in every clinical storehouse.

5.3.7.1 Improving Accuracy

There are no thoughts in robotics systems, they do not get drained, and they never have a slip of consideration. If this seems to be the perfect expert, it was also the thought behind numerous robots that are now found globally in top clinics. Specialists named Waldo can transcend any obstacle between people and machines and execute undertakings with magnificent accuracy, enhanced strength, and no blade quakes. The human specialist takes an auxiliary, controlling task, however long the commodity is set correctly for the passage through the process. As focused on miniature robots, which go precisely where they are needed and transmit tranquilizes locally or even do the miniature medical treatment, such as unclogging veins, astonishing precision often comes as focused miniature robots.

5.3.7.2 Precise Diagnosis

The accurate intensity of AI, assured by InData Labs specialists, lies in identifying designs by considering medical care reports and other details that reflect various situations. Many instances can be verified by the device and associations between many parameters can be searched, some of which are not documented in clinical flow study. So far, studies have shown that robotics frameworks can equal and even outperform the best experts in some zones. For example, an endoscopic system from Japan steadily detects malignant colon growth and is 86% effective. However, this is not as amazing as IBM Watson, which has just reached 99% imprint in the conclusion of malignant development.

5.3.7.3 Remote Treatment

During the 1990s, the most significant proposal to use a robot for therapeutic uses remotely came from DARPA, but correspondence networks were unable to provide real aid in war zone fighters' care. Present rules for 4G and imminent 5G have made this a concern in the past. DARPA tends to support these efforts, but up to this point, it seems that automated medical processes require human Assistance for cleanliness purposes and other activities, leaving things more muddled and not monetarily realistic.

5.3.7.4 Augmenting Human Abilities

Some healthcare machines, regardless of clinical personnel, support patients. Exoskeleton robots, for instance, will allow deadened patients to walk again and be free from supervisors. A genius prosthesis is another utilization of creativity. These bionic appendages have sensors that make them more sensitive and accurate now and then than the first body pieces, adding the possibility of covering them with bionic skin and interfacing them with the person's muscles.

5.3.7.5 Supporting Mental Health and Daily Tasks

Human skills, such as allowing weakened or older adults to feel less desolate, may be exercised by administration robots. Conversational and helpful robots will help these patients stay optimistic, advise them to take their medication, register temperature, circulatory strain, and sugar levels quickly daily. They are equivalent to actual aids and accompany employed in character and slant inquiry skills, useful to discouraged patients.

5.3.7.6 Auxiliary Robots

There is much work in a medical clinic, and professionals should use any support. Medical personnel and clinical faculty may learn from robots' assistance, such as Vigilant Robotics' Moxi robot. This robot deals with replenishment, stuffing, and cleaning so that medical caregivers can devote more resources and provide a human touch to patients while leaving the granulation to the system (RBR Staff, 2019).

5.3.8 CHATBOTS

The lack of expert staff has affected conveying a superior result for patients, and manual cycles in this area have intensified the difficulties. Medical services industry pioneers are going to a broad scope of innovation arrangements, and of them, a broadly embraced are clinical chatbots. If the medical services association's chief, you would very much want to execute clinical chatbots to rearrange your medical care difficulties and improve patient consideration (Hakuna matata tech, 2020). Chatbots can uphold clinical groups by helping their everyday caseloads. In the wake of breaking down the patient information, bots can recommend an online conversation with a clinician instead of visiting their virtual office. In its quintessence, the chatbot innovation is utilized in clinical settings vows to facilitate clinical experts' overload. Also, AI chatbots can improve the supplier's capacity to analyze reliably and precisely. That way, suppliers will likewise have the option to convey care to more patients. Different advantages of utilizing bots are a superior association of patient pathways, moment help in crisis circumstances or emergency treatment, and prescription administration, offering less complicated clinical issues. A chatbot specially designed for the needs of a clinical focus could allow patients to book their arrangements in a moment while never engaging with a human expert or assistant. Medical care providers are now updating bots that help patients verify their side effects and recognize their condition from their homes' comfort. A chatbot will have a point-by-point record of the symptoms pursued and help survey the results of the prescription approved by the managers (Krzysztof, 2020).

5.3.9 ALEXA

The vocalize helped from the Amazon has become productive to the directions of peoples life and interesting working areas in following not too much years' service providers expertise victims likewise medicines expertise used Alexa into the up profession vocalize introducing such as Alexa energize resemblance in between healthcare providers, and the victims authorize people living with diabetes to handle their solution successfully. AWS and the company MERCK and co. Inc started the Alexa diabetes competition with 250,000 US price pot well pepper revolved to the victor in 2018, followed by a professionally striving and

Alexa-based improvement phases to treat diabetes using sugar pod. For example, type 2 diabetes, Alexa helps patients with diabetes control their treatment and seek progress communications, demonstrating how Alexa can be carried out to change tenacious sick individuals.

5.3.9.1 Enhancing Clinic Interrelationships

One of the recently developed Los Angles Aiva uses an Alexa authority program to support victims exploring entertainment with participants such as nurses and home managers. The survivor may ask Alexa to turn either on or off the TV for such a program. Turn the channel to contact the attendant to seek emergency assistance using their mobile phones to aggregate victims, and too many researchers agree that this communicative device will withdraw survivor isolation.

5.3.9.2 Handling Blood Pressure Alexa

By the period of life books so difficulty one of famous clinical devices industries Omron has introduced a watch called "heart guide" a device that can be used to measure blood pressure and convey the readings via Alexa experience.

5.3.9.3 Deducting Wait Duration

Clinics unauthorized Alexa experience employing which victims contacts details for specific departments utilizing this Alexa experience can be able to rescue the period and difficulties via apprise victims regarding the waiting period in every health setting or Sickbay. It assists the victims to get on time and protect critical conditions (RBR Staff, 2019).

5.3.10 BIG DATA

Big data is changing how we break down, use, and oversee information in each industry. Medical services are a promising venture where it may be executed to evade preventable illnesses, improve personal satisfaction, lessen therapy expenses, and gauge epidemics episodes. Health experts can gather a considerable measure of information and locate the best methodologies to utilize the information. It can have positive and life-saving consequences using Big Data in health care. It has gotten more straightforward with arising advances to gather necessary medical services information and convert it into significant experiences to give better care. Well-being experts can forecast and solve a problem before it gets late by using data-driven pieces of information.

We see how enormous information can be utilized in medical care and what advantages it gives.

5.3.10.1 The Expectation of Patients for Strengthened Staffing

Usually, emergency services change operator faces a challenge with the number of employees they bring on board at a given time. On the off chance that a chief keeps an excessive number of laborers, you may have the danger of undesirable work expenses and assets. On the contrary, they have to have a few staff will still create consequences in helpless client treatment that can be more detrimental for the patient's well-being. Big Data can answer this dilemma. Input from a large cluster of outlets should be used for standard output, and the number of patients may be anticipated at the medical center or hospital on an hourly basis. In Paris, four clinics essential for the Assistance Publique-Hôpitaux de Paris have utilized an assortment of sources like 10 years of emergency clinic affirmation records to give every day, and hourly expectations of the number of patients are relied upon to be at the medical clinic at a particular time. In this manner, gathering information and utilizing it to find examples to anticipate conduct can boost workers' staffing by foreseeing patients' confirmation rates.

5.3.10.2   Alerting in Real Time

Furthermore, constant cautioning is vital for critical data investigation in the medical care sector. Clinics use professional decision making tools to investigate clinical knowledge on the spot and furnish wellness specialists with counsel to help them decide on informed decisions. Wearable gadgets are used to persistently capture and transfer the patient's well-being data to the cloud. For example, if a patient's heartbeat spikes suddenly, the framework sends an ongoing signal to the expert that will then be able to attempt to get the pace down and hit the patient. Since IoT devices create a significant data metric, performing insight will help health practitioners decide on meaningful choices and gain continuous caution.

5.3.10.3   Informed Strategic Planning Utilizing Health Data

Massive information in medical services encourages vital arranging. Medical care directors can break down the after-effects of patients' exams in different socioeconomics gatherings. They will also discover variables that prevent patients from taking medication. To create heat maps based on explicit problems such as persistent diseases and population growth, the University of Florida used free global health information and Google Maps. Subsequently, data from emergency providers may also be used to arrange knowledgeable practices.

5.3.10.4   Preventing Human Errors

Typically, experts have been found to either aid in the general dispatch of an alternative substance or inadvertently endorse an off-base medication. Big data can be utilized to diminish such mistakes by dissecting endorsed medication and client information. Prescription data gathered from various clinical experts can be observed utilizing the big data medical care instrument. The product can hail up medicine botches made by any doctors and help save numerous lives (Gordon & Catalini, 2018).

5.4   BENEFITS OF DIGITAL TRANSFORMATION IN HEALTH CARE

5.4.1   BETTER SERVICES FOR PATIENTS

Like whatever another industry means on the way to digital change, medical care is patient (customer)-focused. The execution of various advancements will allow making treatment more customized. The unique methodology is in every case that is better than following expected proposals that probably will not work now and again.

5.4.2 BETTER ANALYSIS

The utilization of such innovations as AI or ML offers occasions to examine information viably and speedily than individuals can do. Likewise, these advancements limit messes up, hence improving staff efficiency.

5.4.3 BETTER ORGANIZATION

On account of Cloud computing and other digital instruments, all the information could be digitalized. It permits speedy admittance to clinical records that allow specialists to settle on choices successfully and give more effective treatment. Also, wearable gadgets could caution both patients and specialists if there should be a crisis in call the rescue vehicle or ambulance.

5.4.4 BETTER TIME MANAGEMENT

The implementation of different digital solutions into the healthcare field saves much valuable time. This is how different lives could be saved when we have, for example, every minute of everyday association with clinical staff.

5.4.5 BETTER ENVIRONMENT FOR DOCTORS

The advancements empower admittance to much information; they give better correspondence and give essential data to the exploration. More significant exploration that specialists could bring about better treatment leads us to the main advantage in our rundown, better administrations for the patients (Hakuna matata tech, 2020).

5.5 CHALLENGES IN DIGITAL TRANSFORMATION

Regulation and Legal Compliance: Guidelines can compel mechanical advancement, especially in intensely managed industries, similar to medical care. The more prohibitive the guidelines, the more troublesome it is to exploit innovative advances.

The Healthcare Industry's Complexity: A medical services environment is significantly more perplexing than any industry. It comprises an assortment of gatherings, factors, and clashing interests—security, HIPAA consistency, client requests, information protection, worker needs, costs, etc.

Dynamic Customer Expectations: Customers need satisfaction and command over their health care or medical care. In the present digital commercial market, they genuinely anticipate it. Simultaneously, they require more command over their information and their protection.

Skill Sets: As referenced, numerous associations believe their laborers to be more digitally developed than the association itself. Notwithstanding, a more granular perspective on this point uncovers a more nuanced issue—as medical care turns out to be more digital, the requirement for specific mechanical aptitudes will increment.

Culture: To get by in the digital period, hierarchical societies ought to turn out to be more digital, more inventive, and more open to change. Similarly, as with some other change ventures, change activities are mind-boggling, long-haul issues (Friedrichsen & Mühl-Benninghaus, 2013).

5.6 CONCLUSION

It is clear from the above discussion that digital solution contributes significantly to the development of healthcare and pharma companies as more organizations have begun to put resources into the advanced digital technique and digital arrangements. The e-healthcare field is just stepping into the heading of computerized change; few nations outrace others, yet at the same time, we cannot consider this wonder a world-wide one. However, because of the accessible advanced medical care innovation that is continually improving and redesigning, we may see another picture of medical ser-vices in the forthcoming years, more proficient and practically perfect. Progressive change or digital transformation is a continuous cycle, and new patterns are arising in the medical services industry as time passes. When you seek digital transformation in medical care, you need to think past the innovation expected to drive development.

REFERENCES

Apple Inc. (n.d.). Augmented reality: Apple developer. Apple.Com. Retrieved December 29, 2020, from https://developer.apple.com/augmented-reality.

Elton, J., & O'Riordan, A. (2016). *Healthcare Disrupted: Next-Generation Business Models and Strategies.* John Wiley & Sons, Hoboken, NJ.

FPFIS team. (2013, May 15). Strategic intelligence monitor on personal Health systems phase 2 (SIMPHS 2) market developments: Remote patient monitoring and treatment, telec-are, fitness/wellness & mHealth. Europa. Eu. https://ec.europa.eu/jrc/en/publication/eur-scientific-and-technical-research-reports/strategic-intelligence-monitor-personal-health-systems-phase-2-simphs-2-market-developments.

Friedrichsen, M., & Mühl-Benninghaus, W. (Eds.). (2013). *Handbook of Social Media Management: Value Chain and Business Models in Changing Media Markets* (2014th ed.). Springer, Berlin. https://www.springer.com/gp/book/9783642288968.

Google.Com. Retrieved December 29, 2020, from https://get.google.com/tango/.

Gordon, W. J., & Catalini, C. (2018). Blockchain technology for healthcare: Facilitating the tran-sition to patient-driven interoperability. *Computational and Structural Biotechnology Journal, 16,* 224–230.

Hakuna matata tech. (2020, November 11). Digital transformation in healthcare 2020-trends & benefits. Hakunamatatatech.com. https://www.hakunamatatatech.com/our-resources/blog/digital-transformation-in-healthcare-technology-trends-and-benefits/.

HCL Technology Q&A. (n.d.). Digital transformation in the healthcare industry? Hcltech. Com. Retrieved December 29, 2020, from https://www.hcltech.com/technology-qa/digital-transformation-healthcare-industry.

Innovative Architects. (n.d.). CLOUD computing services for the healthcare indus-try. Innovativearchitects.Com. Retrieved December 29, 2020, from https://www.innovativearchitects.com/KnowledgeCenter/industry-specific/healthcare-and-cloud-computing.aspx.

Jayaraman, P. P., Forkan, A. R. M., Morshed, A., Haghighi, P. D., & Kang, Y. (2020). Healthcare 4.0: A review of frontiers in digital health. *Wiley Interdisciplinary Reviews: Data Mining and Knowledge Discovery, 10*(2). doi: 10.1002/widm.1350.

Krzysztof, M. (2020, May 5). Chatbots in healthcare: Benefits, risks, and use cases. Codete. Com. https://codete.com/blog/chatbots-in-healthcare/.

Kuo, T.-T., Kim, H.-E., & Ohno-Machado, L. (2017). Blockchain distributed ledger technologies for biomedical and health care applications. *Journal of the American Medical Informatics Association: JAMIA*, *24*(6), 1211–1220.

Microsoft HoloLens. (n.d.). Microsoft.Com. Retrieved December 29, 2020, from https://www.microsoft.com/en-us/hololens/commercial-build.

RBR Staff. (2019, May 29). 6 ways AI and robotics are improving healthcare. Roboticsbusinessreview.com. https://www.roboticsbusinessreview.com/health-medical/6-ways-ai-and-robotics-are-improving-healthcare/.

Reddy, M. (2020, June 19). Digital transformation in healthcare in 2020: 7 key trends. Digitalauthority.Me. https://www.digitalauthority.me/resources/state-of-digital-transformation-healthcare/.

Takyar, A. (2020, May 6). The impact of digital transformation in healthcare. Leewayhertz. Com. https://www.leewayhertz.com/digital-transformation-in-healthcare/.

TD_Madison. (2020). Radiology management, ICU management, healthcare IT, cardiology management, executive management. https://healthmanagement.org/c/healthmanagement/issuearticle/the-future-of-augmented-reality-in-healthcare.

The Medical Futurist. (2017, September 5). HoloLens review: Mixed reality in healthcare: The medical futurist. Medicalfuturist.Com. http://medicalfuturist.com/mixed-reality-healthcare-hololens-review/.

Vial, G. (2019). Understanding digital transformation: A review and a research agenda. *Journal of Strategic Information Systems*, *28*(2), 118–144.

Wright, D., & Androuchko, L. (1996).Telemedicine and developing countries. *Journal of Telemedicine and Telecare*, *2*(2), 63–70.

Yoon, H.-J. (2019). Blockchain technology and healthcare. *Healthcare Informatics Research*, *25*(2), 59–60.

6 Modernizing the Health Insurance Industry Using Blockchain and Smart Contracts

Ali Akbar and Abdullah Mohammad Ali Khan
Jamia Hamdard

CONTENTS

6.1 INTRODUCTION

The concept of insurance is based on the interaction between the insurer (company that guarantees payment for some undetermined future event) and the policyholder, who agrees to pay small amounts or token payments to the insurance company to keep himself protected from future uncertain events (Outreville, 1998). Automobile and health insurance are the most common type of services available, and they make up the majority of the insurance sector.

Research has shown that growth in the health sector directly affects the economic development of the country. Countries like the USA and UK, which have a high Human Development Index, have invested huge amounts of resources in their health sector (United Nations Development Programme, 2019). In these countries, health insurance plays an important role in providing affordable healthcare to all. However, it has been observed that health insurance has been ineffective in penetrating the less privileged section of the society.

The key stakeholders in the insurance industry include the hospitals, insurance company, and the beneficiary. They interact with each other through a complex network of codependent and data-intensive work environments (FICCI and PWC, 2020).

Our objective throughout this chapter has been to minimize the complexity of the insurance industry and – in the process of doing that – make it more secure and accessible to all. In this chapter, we will talk about the health insurance industry and how technologies like blockchain can help us automate and scale the present working processes. We begin by understanding the health insurance industry and its working. From there, we introduce the concept of blockchain and smart contracts. We go through all the available frameworks and resources that can be used in achieving our objective and settle on the most appropriate for our problem. We will analyze the advantages and the possible obstacles we face while implementing our solution. Later on, we will talk about Estonia and its healthcare system which adopted the blockchain technology, and we conclude with our hopes and future research topics related to blockchain.

6.2 LITERATURE REVIEW

It has been more than a decade since Satoshi Nakamoto (anonymous person/group) came up with the paper on Bitcoin and solved the problem of maintaining the order of transactions and avoiding double counting (Nakamoto, 2008). Bitcoin used the concept of grouping the transactions into fixed-size containers called blocks. The miners were held responsible for connecting the blocks in a chronological sequence, and each block would contain the hash of the previous block to maintain sequential insertion and detail lookup (Crosby et al., 2016). This way the blockchain would keep a registry of all the transactions on the network and keep the data stable and secure. The characteristics that make blockchain suitable to replace traditional business processes are its transparency, robustness, auditability, scalability, and security (Christidis & Devetsikiotis, 2016).

The importance of blockchain can be verified by the sudden explosion of cryptocurrencies and their acceptance as a legal form of exchange (CoinMarketCap, 2017). Alternate cryptocurrencies include Ripple (Schwartz et al., 2014), Ethereum (Wood, 2014), etc. Furthermore, the applications of blockchain have transcended to areas such as insurance and supply chain with the introduction of smart contracts. They were first introduced by Szabo (1994) as a "computerized transaction protocol that executes the terms of a contract" (Szabo, 1994), which gives us the ability to translate contractual clauses to actionable code mitigating external risks and damages. As a direct consequence of this, blockchain technology is becoming increasingly mainstream and has a high research potential (Zhao et al., 2016). In this chapter, we will focus on blockchain and its application in the field of health insurance. Healthcare companies are ready to invest in setting up the blockchain infrastructure required for it to succeed. Properties like transparency and auditability can be of great use in the healthcare industry. Blockchains use cases in the insurance industry include sales, customer identification, underwriting, claims processing, and reinsurance (Cognizant, 2017; KPMG International, 2017). For example, insurers in Europe have launched the B3i-a blockchain industry initiative for exploring how it helps in accelerating gains in the insurance industry. Following are some blockchain-based applications in the insurance industry (Mckinsey Company, 2016; Nath, 2016).

6.3 HEALTH INSURANCE

6.3.1 INTRODUCTION

Health insurance is the insurance to cover whole or part of the medical expenses of an individual. The insurance company calculates the amount of monthly payment or premium (a routine payment option) the person has to give, by calculating the risk factor after assessing the health risk. After paying the premium, the insurance company then helps in paying for the health benefits availed or covered under the insurance agreement. A health insurance can be renewable or even be valid for a lifetime.

Following are terminologies that the reader should be familiar (Politi et al., 2013):

Premium: The monthly payment which has to be made for the insurance provider.

Deductible: The amount of money needed to be paid to the insurance provider before it starts covering your bills.

Coverage Limit: Some insurance providers have a set limit to which they will help in the bills.

In-Network Provider: Some insurance companies have quid pro quo with the health care provider. The insurance provider may have a special discounted rate or offers when the patient goes to the specified health care provider. This is widely seen in countries like the United States of America.

Out-of-Network Provider: Some health care centers do not accept health insurance from a particular insurance provider as they are not in contractual agreement as in an In-Network Provider. In these types of situations, the patient has to pay the full medical bill without the help of insurance.

6.3.2 PRESENT STATE OF HEALTH INSURANCE AROUND THE WORLD

Figure 6.1 compares the social/government and private healthcare coverage in different countries. Countries like the UK, Australia, Norway, Netherlands, Switzerland, and Spain have universal healthcare insurance, hence 100% of the infrastructure is supported by the government; whereas in countries like USA, India, and South

Health Insurance Coverage in Countries

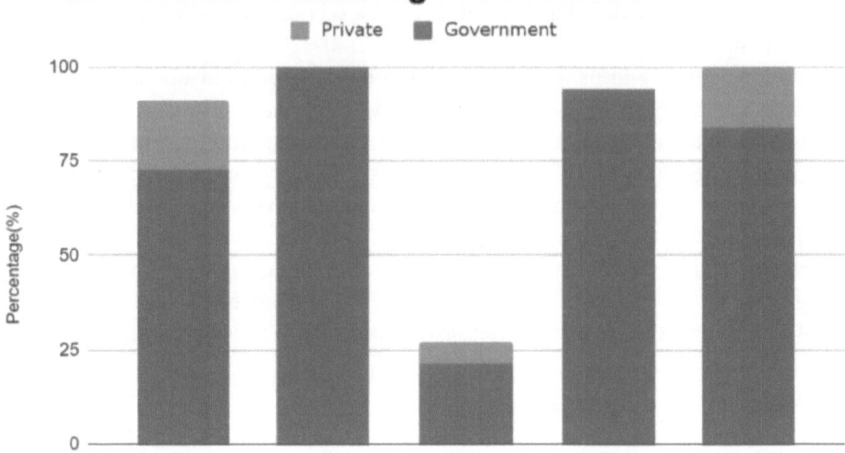

FIGURE 6.1   Health insurance coverage in countries (USA, UK, India, Estonia, South Africa).

Africa, we have both the private and public enterprises playing a crucial role in the insurance system.

Human Development Index is a statistical index computed by incorporating factors such as life expectancy, education, and outreach per capita income variables (Sagar & Naja, 1998). Its range lies between 0 and 1 where unity describes a perfect country and economy, and scores closer to zero reflect an image of underdevelopment and diminishing economy. Table 6.1 gives us the HDI scores of different countries.

Pearson correlation between HDI and insurance coverage of the five countries taken above comes out to be 0.79774. Pearson correlation is a statistical coefficient that measures linear dependencies between two variables, and it is a bivariate measure (Obilor & Amadi et al., 2018). Its value lies in the interval of $(-1, 1)$. -1 denotes negative correlation or inverse relationship, i.e., one variable trend upward while the other trends downward; $+1$ denotes positive correlation; and 0 denotes no correlation. We can say that economic indicators like HDI or GDP are positively correlated with whether the country provides universal healthcare to their citizens or not. Hence we can say that health insurance plays a crucial role in the development and well-being of a country and its citizens. However, it requires a massive amount

TABLE 6.1

HDI of Countries

Countries	Human Development Index (HDI)
USA	0.797
UK	0.845
India	0.647
Estonia	0.882
South Africa	0.705

of computer infrastructure to host consumer data for every individual within the country. Through this chapter, we will describe how blockchain technologies can bridge the gap between the infrastructural challenges and data privacy issues and come out as a common solution for hosting publicly distributed shared data.

6.3.3   HEALTH INSURANCE IN INDIA

A 2014 survey found out that 80% of Indians are not covered in any type of insurance. It is said that it is growing. Yet the government's budget allotted to the health sector still remains comparatively less than other BRICS countries (Times of India, 2018).

India's National Health Programme or Rashtriya Swasthya Bima Yojana, introduced in 2008, was lauded by the World Bank and the UN. However, 12 years later, the condition of the program is far from being laudable. As of 2018, 12 states did not have any central or state health insurance. Even the RSBY had problems being implemented in hospitals. The number of families being covered under this program has also plummeted. A concerning reason for this can be the political agendas of the state government to implement a state-sponsored health insurance program, but this too has failed to come to fruition.

However, the insurance is not only provided by the government. The private market is also a culprit for the slow growth of the Indian insurance sector. These private insurance companies look for profit maximization and cater to the need of the affluent.

The government needs to prioritize bringing an affordable health care plan to the poor and make sure it reaches everyone. In 2018, GoI launched the ambitious Ayushman Bharat – Pradhan Mantri Jan Aarogya Yojana (PMJAY, 2018), which provides health coverage to 40% of the population.

6.4   BLOCKCHAIN AND SMART CONTRACTS

6.4.1   INTRODUCTION

A blockchain, as in its name, is a chain of blocks containing information. A distributed ledger is maintained by network nodes, recording transactions executed between nodes. The data entered in the blockchain is immutable and made available to the public. The concept of blockchain was made popular by the invention of Bitcoin in 2008 by Satoshi Nakamoto. It is a cryptocurrency based on the concept of blockchain, making sure that the centralized control of the bank can be eliminated. The transaction done would be transparent and available to all in a network of computers called nodes. These nodes have a local copy of the public blockchain. One block of this public blockchain consists of a list of transactions completed, a transaction counter which keeps track of the number of transactions, and the most important part, the header.

The header consists of a few things including the hash of previous block, version, timestamp, merkle root, difficulty, and the nonce (Yang et al., 2019). All of this information is then passed through a SHA256 cryptographic hash that generates a 256 bit or 32-byte unique signature of the block which becomes its hash (Selvakumar & Ganadhas, 2009). This hash will be included in the next block also. When the new block is created, it is pushed to all the nodes to update their local copies of the blockchain.

However, to update public blockchain with a common and valid block, a consensus mechanism had to be devised. For this, Satoshi Nakamoto implements a proof-of-work mechanism proposed by Cynthia Dwork in 1993 (Dwork & Naor, 1992).

A proof-of-work mechanism is a computational puzzle available to everyone for solving. The answer to the puzzle is the hash of the block where a group of transactions will be stored. The person solving this puzzle has to validate all the transactions and find the hash of the next block. The first one to solve this puzzle receives some Bitcoin as a reward. This is famously known as Bitcoin mining. Mining is a computationally expensive activity and involves the use of high-end hardware resources.

A smart contract is a digital, self-executing contract that is usually saved on a blockchain (Alharby et al., 2019; Idrees et al., 2021). A smart contract is executed when it receives the information that the set conditions have been fulfilled. The agreement between the two parties is coded into the source code, thus it simplifies the complexity of words. A smart contract provides reduced contract execution cost and improves quality and efficiency.

Ethereum has introduced smart contracts which run on Ethereum blockchain (Buterin, 2014). It is a type of Ethereum account that can send transactions over the network. To use smart contracts, you must know how to code and save it on the blockchain. Ethereum has introduced Solidity and Vyper, two developer-friendly programming languages to write a smart contract.

6.4.2 Public, Private, and Consortium Blockchains

Public: In a public blockchain, we can have any individual to verify blocks of transactions. It is distributed publicly to anyone with an internet connection. The participants of this network remain anonymous and permissionless. The security mechanism implemented in a public blockchain can be proof-of-work or proof-of-stake.

Private: Private blockchains can be assessed by a single organization or a limited number of participants. They are made to cater very specific needs of the company who have full control over its functioning and can be leveraged for business purposes. The participants of this network are known entities who are asked to perform specific functions. It has a high-level security based on the fact that it contains pre-approved participants and uses multi-party consensus algorithms.

Consortium/Permissioned: These blockchains are similar to private blockchains, and the difference lies in the fact that they can have multiple stakeholders controlling their processes instead of one single organization. It has levels of permission levied on the network based on trust. Special participants are given privileged rights in the system.

Public blockchains are slow when compared with private and consortium based as they are light and generally contain fewer nodes (Mohan, 2019).

6.4.3 Blockchain Frameworks

Blockchain applications can be practically implemented on Ethereum and Hyperledger. Both of these platforms are different in their own way.

Ethereum is a decentralized open-source blockchain platform that is capable of running smart contracts. The indigenous currency associated with Ethereum is the Ether, and it has the second-highest market cap behind Bitcoin. It was founded in 2013 by Vitalik Buterin. It uses the POW concept as its consensus algorithm and is programmed in Golang and Python. It uses Solidity programming language for implementing smart contracts.

Hyperledger is an umbrella project for blockchain-based tools by the Linux Foundation. The frameworks which can be found under the Hyperledger project are Hyperledger Fabric, Iroha, and Sawtooth. It is supported by organizations like IBM and Intel. Chaincode is used in Hyperledger Fabric to provide infrastructure and designing of smart contracts permissible.

Hyperledger uses Practical Byzantine Fault Tolerance as its consensus mechanism, which has been used frequently in modern distributed systems. Miguel Castro and Barbara Liskov proposed Practical Byzantine Fault Tolerance in 1999 (Castro & Liskov, 1999). It is a way to reach consensus even among faulty nodes.

The PBFT states that as long as the number of the faulty nodes is less than one-third of the total number of nodes in the system, the system will reach a consensus. It is used in the case of asynchronous internet and helps in optimization.

One of the nodes in the system is appointed as the leader, and the rest become the backup nodes. The client sends a request to the leader node to start service. The leader node then broadcasts the message to other backup nodes. Then the client waits for replies. If there are enough honest nodes available, then they will reach an agreement with a majority. The leading node keeps changing after every protocol. By this way, they reach consensus to update the blockchain.

PBFT is useful when the number of nodes is small. It becomes complex and difficult to scale in a large network as each node has to talk to each other. On the other hand, the power and hardware resource consumption of proof-of-work can be eliminated with this algorithm. The final message agreed with all the nodes will be the final step to completing a transaction which eliminates the waiting time in other consensus mechanisms.

Both of these platforms offer different solutions. They are distinguished in Table 6.2.

TABLE 6.2
Difference between Hyperledger and Ethereum

	Hyperledger	Ethereum
Network	Consortium	Public
Consensus	Practical Byzantine Fault Tolerance(PBFT)	Proof of Work (POW)
Language	Go and Java	Go and Python
Maintained by	Linux Foundation	Ethereum Dev. Community
Cryptocurrency	No specific currency	Ether
Smart contract	Chaincode	Solidity

6.4.4 CAPITAL REQUIREMENTS FOR SETTING UP A CENTRALIZED BLOCKCHAIN FOR HEALTHCARE

Setting up a centralized blockchain network would require significant investments in technology, infrastructure, and human resources. But once set up, it would smoothen the insurance process by digitizing health-related information of the citizens of the country. Building such a database would be highly challenging in India as compared to Estonia but it will come with its own set of advantages if deployed successfully.

The Indian Insurance industry is composed of multiple stakeholders such as insurance companies, hospitals, third-party administrators (TPAs), pharmacies, reinsurers, insurance-based techs, and startups. Blockchain could provide an ideal way to exchange information between all the stakeholders and keep the data up to date and secure. Blockchain can automatically collect policy terms and agreements between different parties and execute the actions when the expectations have been met.

Data quality, data standards, protocols, and reliability are crucial at the beginning of a blockchain cycle and need to continuously improve for it to be successful (Idrees et al., 2021).

The first and foremost requirement for building a technology stack is to set up the infrastructure such as data centers for holding the data. Cloud has been a great alternative for storing large amounts of data, and they are provided by large companies like Microsoft and Amazon at a very affordable cost and can be used to store data.

Hospitals and insurance companies need to have a robust mechanism in place for patient registration and claim processing.

Government needs to play an important and prudent role in setting up a national insurance register.

6.5 INTEGRATING BLOCKCHAIN AND SMART CONTRACTS TO HEALTH INSURANCE

Insurances require an up-to-date information on the transactions done in the past. These interactions with the transaction history usually end up taking a lot of time. This leads to a claim delay.

Another issue that needs to be addressed is the security and validity of the documents. There have been many cases where counterfeit documents have been submitted by the person claiming the insurance. These types of frauds are very common in India. To fight off claim fraud, insurance companies go through lengthy amounts of document verification. However, this doesn't eradicate the venality of the people working in the insurance sector, who might be enticed to help these scammers.

The smart contract is available to everyone, making its conditions out in the open. The users can then compare policies and make the best choice. Most of the time, insurance policies are characterized by the company which provides the policy and not the policy itself. This will promote a fair market.

Blockchain and smart contracts are tamper-proof and secure. By introducing blockchain and smart contracts, we not only secure the data of the consumer, but also make fraud detection easier. The information stored on the blockchain is decentralized so it is accessible everywhere. Any suspicious transaction or behavior will be detected easily.

Everything in blockchain is done digitally, so this will automate the insurance industry. Time-taking process like client registration and policy claiming will speed up. In India, more (insert percentage) people are not registered with health insurance. Simplifying the registration process and putting it on the internet will make it accessible to all and will remove the hassle of paying the middle man.

6.5.1 SELECTING A BLOCKCHAIN DEPENDING ON THE TYPE OF APPLICATION AND DATA SOURCES

First and foremost, we need to find out information about our data source, whether we need a central repository of data or will we collect data from multiple databases and then perform some join operations. If we only have a single data source, we can use it as the central database to perform blockchain operations. Applications with multiple data sources are then subdivided based on the basis of whether they would be open to all or restricted to a few participants acting as privileged nodes. The restricted blockchain should then be a consortium blockchain. The open to all blockchain can be then categorized by identifying what is the verifying mechanism deployed. If there is a central authority then we can use a public-permissioned blockchain, otherwise we can use the non-permissioned distributed public blockchain for our application. Ultimately the decision is based on the following three parameters:

Data Source: Single/Multiple
Access Control: To all nodes/to select nodes
Verifying Authority: Central or every node can act as a verifying authority

6.5.2 IMPLEMENTATION OF SMART CONTRACTS IN HEALTH INSURANCE

We propose a framework that involves the use of smart contracts to automate the health insurance industry. Insurance policy will be available as smart contracts, and along with client information, it will be stored in the blockchain. Smart contracts will also allow proposal forms, medical history, declarations, and unique policy terms and conditions including limits/sublimits to be stored electronically for every type of policy having its own specific requirement. It will also capture the information in an immutable way, making it accessible to relevant stakeholders and preventing any disputes arising from concealing information or false information in a more efficient and faster way.

Customers will basically submit a form that will include relevant documents and medical history to the insurance company. The insurance company will assess the proposal form through artificial intelligence. An underwriting technology will approve the proposal and formulate necessary terms and conditions. Later on, the beneficiary deposits the premium and receives policy documents and related information including the hospital network list.

Claims processing will also work the same way. The beneficiary will submit relevant documents and begin the claims process. The submitted claim will be evaluated

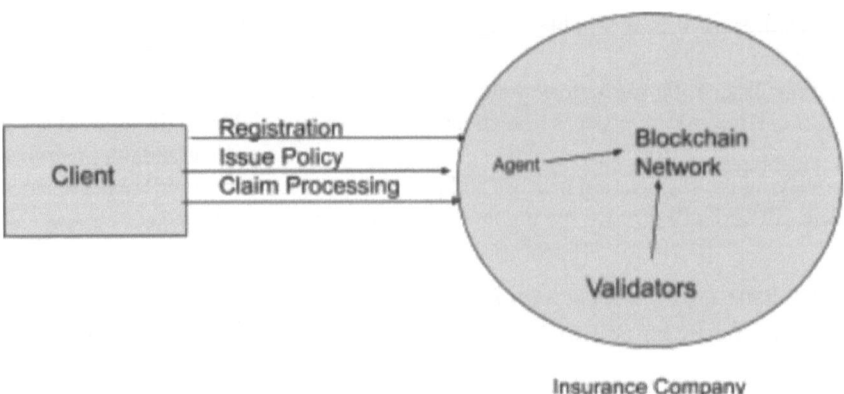

FIGURE 6.2   Client company interaction model.

through artificial intelligence after authorization by the doctor. After the claim is approved, the funds will be transferred directly to the hospital. The customer receives the receipt and other deductions if any.

The validators will validate the claim transaction done between the customer and the insurance company by looking through the history and making sure all the payments are completed and no discrepancies are there. After the validation is completed, the new information will be pushed to the blockchain. This blockchain is a form of permissioned blockchain and its access will be restricted to various stakeholders.

Figure 6.2 depicts the interaction between a customer and the insurance company through the blockchain network. We have the client and insurance company who are interacting with an artificially intelligent agent (wallet, browser plugin) which pushes the data obtained via the transaction to the blockchain. Client has three possible action states to interact which are registration, issuing policy, and claim processing. The role of validators is to verify the transactions and append the blocks to the insurance network.

6.5.3   INSURANCE PROCEDURE IN BLOCKCHAIN

After the implementation of blockchain here's how the insurance company will operate:

  Sale of the Policy: It depends on the medical history, behavioral traits, and financial background of the customer. Private and public health insurances are readily available in the market, and the choice of selecting the policy tends to remain with the customer. The factors that the policy buyer takes into account are affordability, trust with the company, and the number and range of diseases covered under the scheme. Smart contracts will simplify this process.

  Underwriting (Insurer): Rule-based underwriting with immutable and approved guidelines which can be viewed in the smart contract agreement on the blockchain. Mapping the policy data to specific users and offering customized pricing.

Insurer-Hospital Agreement: The insurer and the hospital agree on an arrangement provided they have in place. Tariff agreements and packages agreement as well as contract validity have to be agreed upon mutually by the hospital and the insurer

Electronic Health Records: Accessing the customer's digital identity will be easier with:
- KYC details
- Demographic and medical history details
- Nominee information
- Payout bank details.

Claim Processing: Fast and efficient claims by accessing customer-related information through blockchain and using automated customer authentication. Blockchain will ensure that medical professionals always have updated customer records.

Figure 6.3 summarizes the insurance procedure with a small flowchart.

6.5.4 PROS AND CONS

Implementation of blockchain technology will affect the health insurance market in a positive way. It addresses the problems that are crucial for the growth of this industry.

A major problem with the health insurance systems was that they are not scalable and accessible. Blockchain solves the problem by putting everything online and removing the concept of middlemen. This in turn will decrease the cost of buying insurance. Now people would register online with their information stored on the blockchain and browse policies that they want to buy.

Blockchains are accessible worldwide, which means that all the personal information stored can be accessed anytime by authorized parties. This will lead to a faster and low cost of money transfers. The business process of the insurance industry would speed up substantially. The customers would not have to wait for validation and claims processing.

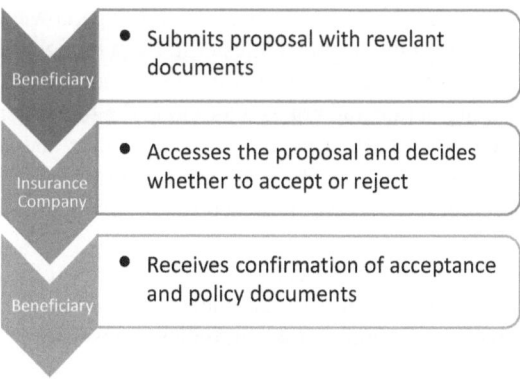

FIGURE 6.3 Insurance procedure using smart contracts.

Blockchains are known most commonly for their security and immutability. Data stored on the blockchain cannot be altered. All transaction history is stored with respect to time, and any false issue claims will be intercepted immediately. This will help in fighting insurance fraud.

Another complaint by the customers was that most of the policies are complex and difficult to comprehend. Smart contracts make the policy conditions transparent and easy to understand at the time of transaction.

There are a lot of advantages to switch to a blockchain-based system in the health insurance sector. However, a few limitations of blockchain technology hinder its chances of being adopted. It becomes risky to implement this without addressing the problem.

The biggest obstacle standing in the way of blockchain automation is the scalability factor. Blockchain, as shown by Bitcoin, is a very hardware expensive technology. To keep it running smoothly, miners use expensive hardware that use up a lot of electrical resources. Bitcoin mining alone takes up to 45 Terawatt of power, which is equivalent to the total power consumed by Austria. This brings the question if it is environment friendly or not. Until and unless we can present an eco-friendly solution to this problem, it will be tough to implement.

If we were to scale it to a country like India which has a population of more than 1.3 billion people, the amount of transactions per day would be unimaginably large. Even though blockchain-based cryptocurrency is faster than most banks, they are handling only a small number of transactions at a time. We have yet to see how blockchain performs on a large scale. Researchers have started to formulate a robust consensus mechanism suitable for large-scale blockchain implementation. Proof-of-stake is one such kind of effort. However, its implementation in Ethereum has to prove its efficiency.

Another issue is the space. Where will the local copies of the blockchain exist and in what form. If we propose to put the whole country's health record information online, we have dedicated data storage facilities available to cater to its need. As for the immutability of the blockchain, if any user gets his or her credentials wrong then it would be difficult to update it.

Blockchain is an efficient solution to some extent, but it's still in its development stage. An average person needs to have some programming knowledge to understand it and would have to spend a lot of time to master it. Even though the volatility of the cryptocurrency market is turning new heads in the direction of blockchain, people only see this as a trading option and not as a tool to make life easier.

Blockchain is secure but it won't be able to stop hackers and crackers to find a way to get into it and manipulate it. Bugs in smart contracts could be exploited by these hackers. Ethereum, in 2016, was attacked by these bug hunters and they stole ~$60 million.

Another blow to the future of blockchain is the success of other technologies which do not have extensive resource requirements. This doesn't help the cause and may turn some people away thinking it is unreliable or unsecure.

6.6 ESTONIA'S DIGITAL HEALTH DATABASE

Estonia has successfully implemented digital solutions to cater to their health infrastructure and insurance needs. Patients and doctors have massively benefitted from the expedient access to health records available at their disposal (Lai et al., 2013).

The Electronic Health Record (e-Health Record) is a nationwide system integrating data from Estonia's different healthcare providers to create a common record every patient can access online. It acts as a central repository of information or a database that hosts information and health records of nearly every citizen of the country. Each and every individual in Estonia, which has visited the hospital premises, will have his/her data getting recorded to the central database which can be then used in the future for medical purposes. Every person is uniquely identified by his electronic ID acting as the primary key of the database. His details are completely secure and can be accessed by restricted nodes only as in the case of permissioned blockchain. It uses blockchain as an integral part to ensure data integration and mitigate attacks and threats to the data structures. Such a database if under the risk of exposure can lead to massive economic and personal losses and hazards. Healthcare data is also used for aggregating national statistical health trends to forecast any epidemic and make sure that the resources employed by the government are utilized to their full potential.

The factors on which the success of the Estonian insurance system relies are discussed in the paper "A case study in blockchain healthcare innovation" (Heston, 2017). Heston points out that the success of this project depends on the ability to keep the database private and safe from maligned usage and the availability of data to hospital services and insurance companies at all times. Estonian government has partnered with private company Guardtime for setting up new innovation clusters and improving current working processes. The application of technology is not limited to healthcare; lately, the government has started to invest in eTaxes, eElections, and eSchools.

The system of centralized healthcare has been widely triumphant in Estonia, but in the life expectancy ranking by the World Health Organization (World Health Statistics, 2016) they were positioned at 40th out of 194 member states. To test the system, we must benchmark Estonia's performance on the WHO metric on a yearly basis for the next 20 years. To adopt a system, we must need to see statistically significant results and improvements in the insurance coverage numbers.

6.7 FUTURE RESEARCH

Blockchain has been a buzzword since Satoshi Nakamoto introduced it with the invention of Bitcoin, a decentralized cryptocurrency that removes the bank as the intermediary. Since then researchers have tried to implement blockchain in different systems of society. Health insurance system is heavily dependent on storing data and validating its authenticity. Blockchain solves this by validating the authenticity of the documents once and storing its digital copy on the blockchain. Once stored in a blockchain, the information becomes accessible from anywhere and is always verified.

However, there are a few obstacles that limit blockchain's success. The biggest one being scalability and energy consumption. There still has to be some research on a better way to reach consensus. One such method that is being tested now is the proof-of-stake. It is a new method of reaching consensus between all the nodes. It may solve the problem of energy consumption by assigning the job of validation randomly to anyone where the probability of getting a chance to be that someone directly depends on how much stake that person has. Ethereum is confident that they can introduce this new technology and replace the existing one.

Engineers are also trying to simplify the process and reduce the complexity. Online wallets and other browser plugins are making blockchain easier for the public to access their data.

Legal regulations are being studied on how to implement blockchain. Smart contracts are yet to be given the green light by the government. Yet, people are positive that the blockchain experiment will be successful like Bitcoin.

Health insurance is just one section of the health sector. Efforts to implement blockchain in health institutions for saving and recording birth date and death date are also in motion. Estonia's success in digitizing its health sector should be an inspiration for other countries to follow. Their blockchain-based medical system is the most cost effective in all of Europe (Ulst, 2007). In the current COVID-19 pandemic, their healthcare system withstood the waves of coronavirus. However, Estonia is a small country with about 1.5 million people. Replicating Estonia's success in a bigger environment is essential for blockchain.

6.8 CONCLUSION

Although the concept of blockchain was introduced in a paper in the 1990s, blockchain has become the technology of the future after the development of Bitcoin. Since then, Blockchain along with machine learning and deep learning has attracted a lot of research and development. IBM, a leader in research of Blockchain, has integrated this technology successfully in different industries. They proudly present their solution in simplifying supply chain management, logistics tracking, healthcare, and other walks of life. IBM has also been working on integrating Blockchain in the insurance industry.

In this chapter, we presented a few of the blockchain framework and proposed our solution with the aforementioned frameworks. Ethereum was chosen because of its ability to integrate smart contracts with it, and we also decided that a private blockchain will be suitable for this industry. Integrating blockchain in the health insurance industry will automate and accelerate the process of registration and claims processing. In doing so it will not only make it accessible to everyone but also secure the data. Digitizing the health insurance procedure will cut a lot of the operational costs and the hassle of the middlemen. Customers would be able to choose their policy not on the basis of company's reputation but on the conditions fulfilled by the policy. In doing so, it will give more power to the customers and break the monopoly of some insurance companies.

Blockchain will also prevent fraud and scams which usually plague the insurance industry. Documents stored on the blockchain cannot be tampered. So, documents will only need to be verified once before pushing them onto the blockchain. However, blockchain's inadequacies are limiting its success in our society. There have to be a few improvements in this technology before it can be integrated everywhere. Not only that, but more people have to be convinced of its qualities so that they can come together to help in proliferating it.

The major issue right now with our solution is the scalability factor. Blockchain has been seen to be a success in a small dataset. When the number and the intensity of the transaction are increased, the network becomes congested and may take a long time to be executed.

A blockchain that is an ultimate solution has yet to be found. Right now, what we have available can become obsolete in the coming 5–10 years. Blockchain industry is evolving at a very fast pace. This gives us hope that a robust solution can be created in the next few years. Another concerning problem is the complexity of blockchain. Average user still finds it very complex and may refuse the blockchain solution. People usually get scared of what they do not understand, so blockchain has to win their trust. There have been consistent efforts to simplify the process or even hide its complexity by the engineers but a solution has yet to be found.

If we are able to tackle these weaknesses and find a viable solution to the above-stated problems, blockchains would then be integrated into today's systems. Insurance company should investigate possible future in the blockchain industry to maximize their reach and security. It will also be favorable to them as blockchain may produce new ways to increase their profits.

REFERENCES

Alharby, M., Aldweesh, A., & van Moorsel, A. (2019). Blockchain-based smart contracts: A systematic mapping study of academic research.

Buterin, V. (2014). A next-generation smart contract and decentralized application platform, https://github.com/ethereum/wiki/wiki/White-Paper.

Castro, M., & Liskov, B. (1999). Practical Byzantine fault tolerance. *OSDI*, 99, 173–186.

Christidis, K. & Devetsikiotis, M. (2016). Blockchains and smart contracts for the internet of things, *IEEE Access*, 4, 2292–2303.

Cognizant (2017). Blockchain: A potential game-changer for life insurance. https://www.cognizant.com/whitepapers/blockchain-a-potential-game-changer-for-life-insurance-codex2484.pdf.

CoinMarketCap (2017). Cryptocurrency market capitalizations, https://coinmarketcap.com/.

Crosby, M., Pattanayak, P., Verma, S., & Kalyanaraman, V. (2016). Blockchain technology: Beyond bitcoin, *Applied Innovation Review*, 2, 6–10.

Dwork, C., & Naor, M. (1992). Pricing via processing or combatting junk mail. *In Annual International Cryptology Conference*, Berlin, Springer, pp. 139–147.

FICCI and PWC (2020). Revamping India's health insurance sector with blockchain and smart contracts. August 2020, https://www.pwc.in/assets/pdfs/healthcare/revamping-indias-health-insurance-sector-with-blockchain-and-smart-contracts.pdf.

Heston, T. (2017). A case study in blockchain health care innovation. *International Journal of Current Research*, 9, 60587–60588. doi: 10.22541/au.151060471.10755953.

Idrees, S.M.; Nowostawski, M.; Jameel, R.; Mourya, A.K. Security Aspects of Blockchain Technology Intended for Industrial Applications. Electronics 2021, 10, 951. https://doi.org/10.3390/electronics10080951

Idrees, S. M., Nowostawski, M., & Jameel, R. (2021). Blockchain-based digital contact tracing apps for COVID-19 pandemic management: Issues, challenges, solutions, and future directions. *JMIR Medical Informatics*, 9(2), e25245.

Zhao, J.L., Fan, S., & Yan, J. (2016). Overview of business innovations and research opportunities in blockchain and introduction to the special issue, *Financial Innovation*, 2(1), 28.

KPMG International (2017). Blockchain accelerates insurance transformation. https://assets.kpmg.com/content/dam/kpmg/xx/pdf/2017/01/blockchain-accelerates-insurance-transformation-fs.pdf.

Lai, T., Habicht, T., Kahur, K., Reinap, M., Kiivet, R., & Van Ginneken, E. (2013). Estonia: Health system review. *Health Systems in Transition,* 15, 1–196.

McKinsey Company (2016). Blockchain in insurance-opportunity or threat? https://www.mckinsey.com/industries/financial-services/our-insights/blockchain-in-insurance-opportunity-or-threat.

Mohan, C. (2019). State of public and private blockchains: Myths and reality, pp. 404–411. doi: 10.1145/3299869.3314116.

Nakamoto, S. (2008). Bitcoin: A peer-to-peer electronic cash system.

Nath, I. (2016). Data exchange platform to fight insurance fraud on blockchain, *IEEE International Conference on Data Mining Workshops, ICDMW*, Barcelona, Spain, pp. 821–825.

Obilor, E.I., & Amadi, E. (2018). Test for significance of Pearson's correlation coefficient.

Outreville, J. (1998). Insurance concepts. In *Theory and Practice of Insurance*. Springer, Boston, MA. doi: 10.1007/978-1-4615-6187-3_8.

PMJAY (2018). PMJAY Link: www.pmjay.gov.in.

Politi, M., Kaphingst, K., Kreuter, M., Shacham, E., Lovell, M., & McBride, T. (2013). Knowledge of health insurance terminology and details among the uninsured. *Medical Care Research and Review (MCRR)*, 71. doi: 10.1177/1077558713505327.

Sagar, A. & Najam, A. (1998). The human development index: A critical review. *Ecological Economics*, 25, 249–264. doi: 10.1016/S0921-8009(97)00168-7.

Schwartz, D., Youngs, N., & Britto, A. (2014). The ripple protocol consensus algorithm. Technical Report. https://ripple.com/files/ripple consensus whitepaper.pdf.

Selvakumar, A.L. & Ganadhas, C.S. (2009). The evaluation report of SHA-256 crypt analysis hash function, *2009 International Conference on Communication Software and Networks*, Macau, pp. 588–592. doi: 10.1109/ICCSN.2009.50.

Szabo, N. (1994). Smart contracts.

Times of India (2018). https://timesofindia.indiatimes.com/business/india-business/12-states-have-no-state-or-central-health-insurance/articleshow/63035172.cms.

Ulst, M. (2007). Overview of the healthcare system in Estonia: A personal view. Accessed 2020. https://healthmanagement.org/c/imaging/issuearticle/overview-of-the-healthcare-system-in-estonia-a-personal-view.

United Nations Development Programme (2019). Beyond income, beyond averages, beyond today: Inequalities in human development in the 21st century (PDF). HDRO (Human Development Report Office), pp. 22–25. Retrieved 9 December 2019.

Wood, G. (2014). Ethereum: A secure decentralised generalised transaction ledger, *Ethereum Project Yellow Paper*, 151, 1–32.

World Health Statistics (2016). Monitoring health for the SDGs, sustainable development-goals. Geneva, Switzerland, World Health Organization, 2016. http://apps.who.int/iris/bitstream/10665/206498/1/9789241565264_eng.pdf.

Yang, X., Liu, J., & Li, X. (2019). Research and analysis of blockchain data, *Journal of Physics: Conference Series*, 1237, 022084. doi: 10.1088/1742–6596/1237/2/022084.

7 Blockchain Technology Applications for Improving Quality of Electronic Healthcare System

Pankaj Bhatt, Suruchi Singh,
Satish Kumar Sharma, and Vipin Kumar
Glocal University

CONTENTS

DOI: 10.1201/9781003141471-7

7.1   INTRODUCTION

Blockchain technology is the transformation of technology. The technology we were talking about would have transformed the healthcare is blockchain. Blockchain can be altered how doctors can approach a patient or casualty details, and how would healthcare investigation occur with the healthcare biological community of interacting organisms (Singh, 2019; Idrees et al., 2021, Idrees et al. 2021).

The central authority (firmly like Google, small commercial business single person) monitored the spread-out ledger of the same blockchain bibliography (Ledger, 2019). In a blockchain, essential thing is a ledger that implements the necessary changes and updates it when all the transactions are recorded among different parties. (Peter & Panayi, 2016). Understanding the results of clinical research and standardization, inability to regenerate the investigation significantly, and medical science that was discovered cannot be regenerated as they were fully bug's (Ioannidis, 2003, 2005; Colhoun et al., 2003). Blockchain technology is regarded as a step for better clarity that allows to build trust between patient and research communities. It ensure to improve clinical research methodology. (Irving & Holden, 2016). Blockchain is a computer treaty which composes cryptography, a modern method to find bibliography, sociocultural legitimate political insurrection and facts information as well as skills establishment, that will be affected by it. The blockchain possess the space checkmate digital best ever unchangeable translucent (Bartling, 2019).

7.2   BLOCKCHAIN REVOLUTION: THE TECHNICAL
IMPLEMENTATIONS

The blockchain aspects were organized via the cryptographic procedure and official agreement. They were famous long ago and had also been elaborated to control the hardware's negligence, e.g., the extensive database (Bartling & Fecher, 2016). In this day, they were employed to supply faith within other time not known condition, and shared existence of blockchain system depends on various separate computers to protect blockchain system and yield the confidence or protection presently yielded by a controller. These computers can be unidentified organizations encouraged to perform so through inherent benefits congenital to the system (e.g., bitcoins Ethereum) (Ethereum Foundation, 2015). They further described central command that the protected computer could be yielded by confidence conditional and self-reliant investigation college (Wisniewska, 2016) or government association; nevertheless, invariance can be done by confidential third-party managers. In the present day, the blockchain-protecting computers cannot change bibliography stockpiles. In the blockchain system, in a unauthoritative character, even if some orders I want them to perform it just supplied cryptographic ability to protect the blockchain even though if the unquestionable quantity of them strikes a balance of bibliography, which has been kept in blockchain system that will turn to be undependable entirely and changeable.

7.3 BLOCKCHAIN IN HEALTHCARE SYSTEM

7.3.1 Current Healthcare System

Healthcare is a type of data-intensive clinical domain in which many data are created, broadcasted, and examined daily. As this data is susceptible to security and privacy spreading, storing a large amount of information is a complicated and challenging task. To focus on the quality of healthcare service means that we are trying our best to provide the patient with superior-level health management (Griebel et al., 2015). However, because of its rules and regulation, the task is becoming much more complicated and lengthy. It is not possible under this process to make the patient healthcare practically. There is a vast difference among peers and providers, which is the main issue or concern to provide quality healthcare services. The middle man in this makes the task more difficult. The first information and data regarding the patient healthcare spread a different level like department, system, etc. That is why it is complicated to find the critical data whenever required. It is not a smooth process as the management of the healthcare ecosystem is in multiple hands. In the field of healthcare and clinical setting, it works with 3S: secure, safe, and scalable data sharing is required to diagnose the combination of clinical decision-making. The technique related to the sharing of data is essential as it allows the clinical practitioners to transfer the patients' clinical information to the authority that is concerned so that quick results can be taken. The information giver and receiver should do the process in the most sensitive and private form so that both of them get correct and complete information about the patient's condition so that necessary steps can be taken.

To get the expert's opinion, the major two domains are e-health and telemedicine; the other two domains are used to transfer the data to the specialist at far-off places (Houston et al., 1999). The information is being transferred through online real-time clinical monitoring or store and forward technology. The government, the provider community, and the healthcare authority are waiting for the new possibilities originated by blockchain. It is being done by the FinTech industry, which has motivated others to do it in the more effective and speculative potential application. The moment is called a utopian moment. The industry should also emphasize establishing blockchain and building the ecosystem partners to form the standard or boost up for implementing it on a large scale for future results. Hyperledger foundation is the best example among the most developing blockchain concerts of the model for the healthcare space. This foundation is an open source that has been formed to create new ideas for cross-industry blockchain technologies. We should know about the hype cycle that has been formed at the blockchain technology and its result in healthcare applications. We can also believe that out of all the cases, the one mentioned is the best at the right degree of adoption among different countries and various healthcare systems (Das, 2017).

7.3.2   Clinical Health Data Exchange and Security

Data exchange is the first topic to study while dealing with blockchain in healthcare. Blockchain helps the health IT system deal with the technological solution facing many challenges that comprise integrity, portable user-owned data, health data interoperability, security, and many other areas. Blockchain allows only that data exchange system to work, which is cryptographically safe and reversed. Reducing the burden and price of data reconciliation helps provide information about the patient related to the past and present. The current participation among data-centric security companies, the Estonian eHealth Foundation and Guardtime, sets an example for blockchain technology. It provides the health record for ~1 million Estonian citizens using KSI, a keyless signature infrastructure. Keeping in mind the difficulty faced by governance structure and data ownership regarding health data exchange with private and public entities, it is impossible to duplicate the Estonian blockchain-secured health record model worldwide (Das, 2017).

Different challenges are faced during this domain. Different critical challenges are faced at practical operations regarding security, safety, and clinical data exchange between research institutions and healthcare organizations. It follows specific processes like sharing data with the agreement, governing the rules, clinical data and its nature, procedures, sensitivity, and ethnic policies (Downing et al., 2017). There is no need for a third party to carry out the transaction to implement the application related to blockchain technology (Git, 2017). The blockchain, with its mechanism, enables the group to provide the information in blockchain architecture (Zheng et al., 2017), removing the risk of security and privacy. The data and privacy are incomplete as the note allows the data to be transferred from one to the other. If there is no third party involved at the time of emergency, the patient has to select more than one representative to collect medical history information (Frankenfield, 2020). This representative will also allow the group of people to find a record of that patient and lead to a data security threat and privacy. There can be blockage if the record is being transferred from one block to another, and the person who receives it has incomplete data. Blockchain network is related to the type of security that is 51% attacks; it can lead to the group of minors that is more than 50% in the blockchain network (Hertig, 2018). It prevents new information after taking permission. If it relates to CoinDesk, five cryptocurrencies are the sufferer of the attack. The patient's record may be so vital that it is not suitable for blockchain (Linn & Koo, 2020).

7.3.3   Pharma Clinical Trials and Population Health Research

Approximately 50% clinical test was undeclared, and researchers frequently did not spread their research outcomes (e.g., almost 90% of tests on clinicaltrial.gov have not outcomes). Blockchain authorized period imprints unchangeable history of the clinical test system, and outcomes can monologue the matter in the future result change detail inquiry and choosy announce. Mainly blockchain based system helps to manage the unknown event between the researchers as well participants with a new ideas in the field of medical research like precision medicine and population health management. (Das, 2017).

7.3.4 BLOCKCHAINS IN ELECTRONIC HEALTH RECORDS (EHR)

In the previous 10 years, the demand for a complete increase in modifying medical health history resulted from health personnel Sickbay and health management types of equipment computerized details make it simple to enter and distribute Likewise, the condition of good and speedy resolution stands even though electronic health history (EHH) was never generated. Electronic health record is not formed to deal will the daily updated records of different institute and patients who spread the information with different institute e.g. situation based on life separates from one with the other providers information. Through this they miss the chance for the past information. (Mandl, 2001; Brandon et al., 1991; Gorman, 2006). Med Rec, a prototype that used different types of blockchain perks and helps to manage the evidence, secrecy, purity, and also shares the data easily. Decentralized Record Management System works on this method. It works in providing the patients with immunable and descriptable history. It allows providing the healthcare information easily among different institute and provider. A predecessor named "metric" used clear-cut blockchain FAQ in handling attestation and concealment integrity and simple distribution of details. Ach acts on a decentralized history control system and allegation to supplied victim EC council; it is on changeable record and makes it easier to meet their particular health management details over various supplier and therapeutic institutes (Ekblaw et al., 2016).

7.3.5 DRUG SUPPLY CHAIN INTEGRITY AND PROVENANCE

When calculated from the industrial point of view it was found that Pharmaceuticals companies suffer a loss of $200 billion worldwide because of counterfeit drug annually. 30% of the drug are regarded as counterfeit and sold in mostly developing countries. . InTouch can aid in bringing evidence in possession of medicine origin at any given a tip in the provide sequence and handle the communication among various victims, for instance, an industry called iSolve LLC is presently functioning together with many pharma/biopharma industries to carry out its modern digital ledger technology (MDLT) blockchain solution to assist medicine to provide sequence honesty (Das, 201).

7.3.6 BLOCKCHAINS IN PHARMACEUTICAL INDUSTRY AND RESEARCH

The pharmaceutical sector is the fastest-growing primary sector at the forefront of healthcare delivery in the pharmaceutical industry. The pharmaceutical sector keeps in mind about safety, security, and validity of the medicinal products and the drugs to be sold to the customers (Mettler, 2016). It also manufactures new drugs that are in demand from different customers. It produces only those products that are beneficial for the patient and make his recovery quicker. In many cases, the drug company faces the risk of finding out the product on a timely basis, which can lead to the severe risk that allows counterfeiters to accommodate the manufacturing and add falls drug into the system. The most common and significant health risk spread in a developing country is the distribution and production of counterfeit drugs (Taylor, 2016).

TABLE 7.1

Various Applications of Blockchain Technology in the Healthcare System

Applications	Summary
Electronic Health Records	A computerized EHR on a disseminated record of a permitted blockchain is ensured with trustworthiness, from the information age phase to the point of information recovery, without human mediation
Clinical Research	Blockchain presents a decentralized, secure structure for any joint data efforts that could occur concerning clinical exploration. With this, information can be safely imparted to gatherings of scientists
Medical Fraud Detection	Blockchain, having the element of being permanent, helps in misrepresentation identification by not permitting any duplication or change in the exchange, and in the long run, permits a direct and secure exchange.
Neuroscience Research	Blockchain, as a development, brings a few open applications consolidating cerebrum increase, a re-order of the mind, and cerebrum thinking. Digitizing an entire human mind requires some medium to store it, and it is here that blockchain advancement raises its head
Pharmaceutical Industry and Research	Blockchain, utilizing its capacity of the definite following, watches out for each phase of the drug store network: The beginning of the medication, its segments, and possession are often distinguished at each stage to keep away from the fashioning/taking of products

Blockchain is the best suitable technology for research, development, and production as it helps to monitor and evaluate the required drugs. It has formed a counterfeit medicine project that helps fight the production of counterfeit drugs (Plotnikov & Kuznetsova, 2018). By using digital technologies, especially in developing countries, there is a need to calculate, evaluate, and enable the supply of pharmaceutical drugs before giving them to the patient. To get protection from counterfeit drugs, a digital drug control system is the best process as a solution that we can think about (Марков, 2018). Pharmaceutical industries have launched a joint pilot project by using DDCS in blockchain to monitor and evaluate the new drugs launched (Sylim et al., 2018). Using this approach makes it possible to find out the location and production (Trujllo & Guillermo 2018), but it also helps remove the fake drug. There should be a guarantee for the safety and security of drugs supplied and given to the customer for consumption. The quality also has to be kept in mind (Plotnikov & Kuznetsova, 2018). As seen in Table 7.1, there are various applications of adopting blockchain to advance biomedical/healthcare research below.

7.3.7 BLOCKCHAIN TECHNOLOGY FOR IMPROVING CLINICAL RESEARCH QUALITY

The two main characteristics of data at the functional level are historicity of the data and inviolability. Blockchain helps to find safety in posterior reconstruction analysis. It helps to arrange all the calculated events in their chronological order (Perez-Marco, 2016). It checks data integrity that refers to validate every transaction cryptographically. This also enables safety, reduces false data, and helps find the correct invention (Gipp et al., 2015). In the second chance, the given data's history and traceability is the technology's primary function that helps blockchain record the time taken. This information is open for all. Anyone can take a copy of the given information (CONSORT, 2010; Chan et al., 2013; WHO Data Set, 2020). Blockchain stores primary and secondary data, Including and excluding criteria are grouped in a data structure at the beginning of the clinical trial. It helps protect from main issues like differences in the plant outcome protocol and the resulted publication, selecting reported outcomes related to reporting the harmful element (Ioannidis et al., 2004; ICH E9 Expert Working Group, 1999; Moher et al., 1999). These issues are shifted on one side and are bias in nature. Before completing the study, there is an urgent need for a statistical analysis plan rather than blindly studying it (Moher et al., 1994; Mulward & Gotzsche, 1996). The data comprises defining the heavy events, adjusting a group of variables, and statistical methods (Sandve et al., 2013). Search teams do not have the exact outcome of the information, so they take the estimated value, which can be bought in some cases (Omenn et al., 2012). To prevent analytical errors, analytical code must be made open for all and shared globally. It focuses on the control version and, at the same time, cannot be prevented from changes in the period. The "git" is used as a code that helps check and analyze its production (Git, 2017).

7.3.8 BLOCKCHAIN TO IMPROVE THE TRUSTABILITY OF CLINICAL TRIALS

Detrimental research practices can occur at any step of a clinical trial, from the beginning of the trial design to the report's end. The biggest challenge related to our times medical is the low productivity of clinical research (Ioannidis, 2005; Mathieu et al., 2009). This issue has many numbers of examples in the scientific literature. The most reappearing issues are lack of data sharing, selected outcomes and swift outcomes. It is concerned with the fact modification that allows the blockchain for the integrity of the events and arranges them in proper chronological order to be adequately traced and improve its productivity (Benchoufi et al., 2017). A clinical trial is also a complex task that can be misused and misconducted. A clinical trial can be protected from the blockchain as it maintains the data's security and privacy. Metadata of a clinical trial is attached through the sources and the software as it is a mandatory task by regulatory authorities. One more process is done through which data analyses can be assessed through the third party without breaking the secrecy and tracing it to reinforce it. The events' transparency index and smart contract-validated workstreams can be built (Graham et al., 2005). The essential evolution that the blockchain-powered repository of a clinical trial is the same as a medical image has its document that is in DCOM format, and it is a confidential format. It is used for search engines and can be reused, and data can be shared and archiving. Architecture choices are very technical and have a figuring effect on the design that has a solution, and are bonded with high-level methodological choices. After practicing, two things can be occupied in public life proof of data and metadata (Cachin, 2016).

Encrypted objects are also referred to as hashes whose unity can be verified. After the concerned party's approval, personal data can be stored on a private blockchain (Jayachandran, 2017). Because of privacy and security, private blocking is more popular. Hyper leisure is an example of the private blockchain. It is unlawful for special needs of hybrid office guarantee and security from a distributor network when private blockchain cannot be void. The hosting can work on the private and public blockchain to communicate quickly, and a solution of the uniform layer is being incorporated. It also helps maintain the state of the system on private and public blockchain (Dai et al., 2018).

7.3.8.1 Problems/Limitations

Inaccuracy is the main problem faced by the clinical research industry when applying the blockchain technology in case of integration, application regulations, and its implementation. The most pharmaceutical organization believes that there is a need to follow it faster than to implement. The primary limitations are as follows:

1. Trust-related issues.
2. There is a reduction of central controlling authority: there is only Uni central organization or state.
3. Limited measurability (Omar et al., 2020).

7.3.9   BLOCKCHAIN IN DRUG TRACEABILITY

Blockchain is a type of network that distributes the data in verified time by the pharmaceutical industries that trace and track the drugs that are shipped and manufactured by the users. The main concern of the healthcare industry is drug counterfeit (Mearian, 2019). It is challenging for the healthcare industry to fix it if it reaches 10%–30% of the drug counterfeit. It not only reduces the cost but can also affect the patient. The value of the counterfeit drug in the market is about $200 billion yearly. China and India are the largest producers of this medicine. This is the main reason of concern and has to be taken care of by using blockchain. This medicine contains different types of ingredients or essential ingredients. Due to this, it is harmful. Blockchain solves this problem by ensuring the traceability of drugs and security. Blockchain mainly adds records to the block. The information is fixed and recorded for verification in the future. That is why they are fixed when the whole supply chain is shifted to the blockchain. This is the best guide given for the blockchain that is used in pharma. The private blockchain is used when required by the hospital information system.

The simple way is to use both public blockchain and private blockchain. This information can be safe and shared publicly before the circulation drug is registered on the concerning blockchain. The drug chain which is not shown in the blockchain may be regarded as fake and unreal. It is used to check the originality of the drugs. In blockchains, different platforms work together. It is easy to find out the drug and increase how the drug is being passed to the retailers and patients (Singh, 2019). A significant number of pharmaceutical ingredients needed in the manufacturing of drugs are imported from outside the country.

Every step from production to drug distribution must follow drug supply chain regulation by law. Many medicines are sensitive and require to be stored in a temperature-controlled environment. However, in the current software, the storage of these cold chains shipping information is done on the centralized databases, which are highly prone to data hacks and can be manipulated (Daue, 2017). That is why it is essential to assign a safe system for the traceability of drugs to overcome counterfeiting. Many steps have been taken by the government worldwide for drug disability. Patients and other stakeholders can easily trace drugs' location in the drug supply chain and verify their legitimacy through a secure drug traceable system (Tian, 2017). At the time of the drug supply chain, when the transaction of drugs keeps changing from different stakeholders, the work of the drug disability system keeps the record of the transaction (Lu & Xu, 2017). For any counterfeit purpose, when the information flows from different stakeholders and patients, the data it provides should be adequate and informative (Li et al., 2017). It should record the drug's security to the required stakeholders for the government's regulations and hold them together. There is a need for the privacy of traceable data in the system as it helps to keep the information safe and secure (Toyoda et al., 2017).

7.3.10 PATIENT DATA MANAGEMENT

The health of the person can get worse with the issue related to health and many others. It means dealing with every patient is very difficult, and that ensures patient data management. Different types of treatment and strategies are being required to deal with different types of patients. For this, complete information about the patient is required. The same type of treatment is not compulsory that it will work on the other patient as well; that is why different patients require a different type of treatment. It helps to get personalized care with patient-centric treatment. If the patient's information is incomplete, then it is also a challenging task for the physician. It can also add the cost for healthcare. This is not safe and is insecure. Doctors these days are also using unsafe ways to share information. Also, the doctors are sharing the information about the patient and their healthcare through the media. This leads to the leakage of information about the patient (Singh, 2019). In this case, blockchain helps to manage the data of the patient. The right professional blockchain also allows keeping the data regarding the patient's health in a proper way. The patient's record is being kept and can be assessed by only the doctor who is using it. It also ensures that the patient has the absolute right to maintain the security of his medical report.

Healthcare organization through API only manages that information about the patient who are not sensitive. It helps to collaborate throughout the system properly. Doctors can also get the data whenever required. After combining with IoT, the researchers can examine the patient's conditions like the vital body part, heartbeat, etc. Blockchain and IoT help to decide a quicker way and can save the life of the patient. The author also explains that healthcare has played an essential role in storing the individual's information. It has significant effects on the lives of the people who can steal this data, and they can sell it to make income, so blockchain helps prevent this task. This is why authors have a form of blockchain-based information preservation framework that helps maintain the data's secrecy.

Ethereum is the platform in which they have presented this data. It helps to get the result in the best and accurate manner. At the time of adding a new patient, it added to the new blockchain at the existing blockchain structure. These blockchains are interlinked with each other and have a suitable network. Every blockchain has a verified time and contains the vital information of the previous block also. The system examines every record properly so that no misuse is done. The blockchain minimizes the risk related to the patient's medical record (Li et al., 2018).

7.3.11 BLOCKCHAIN FOR ELECTRONIC MEDICAL RECORD (EMR) DATA MANAGEMENT

Using the technology of blockchain in the hospital is being tested by several pilot projects worldwide. In the previous year in the United States, Booz, Allen Hamilton consulting has discovered and implemented this blockchain-based pilot platform for helping Food and Drug Administration office by using this technology to manage the data for the person's health. This project has taken place among four hospitals. The project is being done on IPFC to reduce the duplication of the data that include the cloud component with a cryptographic algorithm for creating the sharing of user information (Vahdati et al., 2021). The link is contentious in Europe between the General Data Protection Regulation (GDPR) and blockchain. Blockchain and Healthcare Data Protection in Europe the connection between blockchains and the general data Protection Regulation (GDPR) is relatively dubious.

On the one hand, blockchains appear to speak to a decent arrangement with GDPR (regarding information versatility, for instance, or assent the board, information recognizability, and legal access auditability). Different issues can be recognized (regarding the option to be failed to remember, yet also when the specialized usage through savvy agreements may debilitate the real authority over information through programmed execution). One choice to handle this issue is "dynamic assent the executives", completely by the GDPR arrangement concerning assent (Kaye et al., 2015). Besides, it is considered that "private blockchains", e.g., Enterprise Blockchain, can easily comply with GDPR directives since the transactions of the digital records of the stored information can be modified and erased by private entities or authorities who can own and control this platform, using a particular class of consensus algorithm. A single company or organization from this private blockchain can be used by multiple users guaranteed and agreed upon by the concerned patient. This system works how the company manages the application. Their use in such cases includes public health records owners, healthcare reimbursement providers, and record-keeping by government agencies. This blockchain will have a beneficial impact in the future year and benefit from the policy and its management. Its abilities have also been shown by the European Commission research and innovation program IMI pilot project by the name blockchain-enabled healthcare that is being formed by Novartis whose primary purpose is to maintain the standard like a goal and helps in developing the standard wherever required. The main concern is to enable the service that satisfies the patient. The blockchain system focuses on wearable sensors and medical IoT devices like personal health records (PHR). The complete PHR service trajectory forms the vital source of data that relates to the blockchain service provider. Real-time artificial intelligence (AI) focused on healthcare analytics is being formed on related users like pharmaceutical researchers, payers, physicians, and patients (Dimitrov, 2016; Salah et al., 2019).

7.3.12   BLOCKCHAIN FOR EHR DATA MANAGEMENT

For managing the data of electronic health record (EHR), blockchain technology is essential. Smart contracts can enable the patient by using the token and can share their data related to medical healthcare with the research partners and providers at the desirable cost. For example, Health Wizz is piloting a blockchain- and FHIR-enabled EHR aggregator mobile app, which uses blockchains to tokenize data, enabling patients to securely aggregate, organize, share, donate, and/or trade their personal medical records. One such example is health-wise that focuses on a platform of blockchain that allows FHIR to facilitate EHR aggregator mobile in which blockchain focus on the data linked with tokens, sharing and also enables the patient to give the data with safety, organize and trade the medical records related to the personal health (Healthwizz, 2019). By this method, the patient can keep track of their health medical record as they do it in case of the bank account online to communicate between caregivers and healthcare organization for a better standard of living. Like an EHR Blockchain company, the medical chain is also putting an effort to ensure that the main healthcare agents like laboratories, insurers, doctors, pharmacists, and hospitals get the information about the person's medical record (Medicalchain, 2020). All the interaction should be safe, secure, and transparent, and after this, it is recorded in the ledger of medical chains distributed ledger. The authors have complete faith in the information that is electronically a medical records being shared and it also reduces the cost related to the medical service. Keeping a record of the person's health and medical is quite challenging as the data is not secure. For this purpose, blockchain-based approach is being set up so that the data's security is being maintained. After implementing the electronic medical record, it is secured from misuse and ensures the data's adequacy. The system is not rigid and helps to maintain a transparent audit. One more framework regarding the blockchain is being prepared that focuses on cancer patients. This framework's prototype helps maintain privacy and security and helps store, save, and share the data. The main framework regarding this comprises the database for medical data storage, API, membership service, and nodes. Whosoever is assessing the complete progress of the blockchain has to confirm to the blockchain miners at the time of functioning of membership service. By using the symmetry key, the profile first needs to be confirmed through the user's authorized digital signature, and then it is to be given to the doctor for the different query-cloud server and local database other too sensitive healthcare stored in the database. Cloud server consists of the information that is being put in proper order. The local database consists of information related to cancer patients. All the information related to these two databases is arranged in a proper symmetric key that changes from patient to patient. This is related to the type of control that is being identified for the patient. The authors do the entire check and control to maintain the security and privacy related to the patient medical health record (Yang & Yang, 2017).

7.3.13 BLOCKCHAIN FOR POINT-OF-CARE GENOMICS

According to a blockchain platform company, Timi, the patient information value is calculated as USD 7000 per year (Zajc, 2018). Most mHealth companies focus on personal EHRs and the profile that collect the information through wearable sensors, personal genome, etc., about the patient or own and sell their health data. That is why the consumer companies are providing sequences for DNA for the given time. The company that is providing direct to customer genetic testing service is the most productive. One such company is 23 and Me, which was established in the year 2006. The main concern related to the healthcare industry is to maintain its privacy (Bates, 2018). In the last year, it was shown that this company had sold the customers' data of about 5 million USD 300 million stakes to the pharmaceutical giant Glaxo Smith Kline that only contains exome data. The blockchain has worked in the healthcare-related issue to find a solution for the customers who want DNA test results and want their data to be kept secret (Collins, 2019).They also provide the data to monetize through blockchain-supported providers. For example, the general nebula mix is providing a whole-genome sequence for free. If any user has the sequence of the genome, they can charge the money through that. They can give it in the form of a token to those who require it. The token can, in the future, be used for more tests that can relate to DNA genomes. IO is one more example of blockchain, enabling the customers to store their genome after getting it in the sequence form selectively. The aim of this is to protect the information related to the patient from falling into the wrong hands, and the customers can on their own sell their genetic data if they want to (Genomes.io, 2020).

7.3.14 MEDICAL INSURANCE STORAGE SYSTEM

The main aim of the authors is related to the blockchain-based medical insurance storage system. This is only possible because of credibility and decentralization property. The stakeholders that are related to this are servers, emergency clinics, patients, and insurance agencies. It promises to focus on lawful information that needs CPU and low memory. According to the Ethereum platform, all the information about this has to be checked and then calculated. The system management layer, storage layer, and user layer are the three main layers that the author has kept in mind. System management is the primary layer in which transactions are secured, and it is the central layer. The storage layer is the layer in which all the information is stored correctly for application on the cloud. The user layer comprises the blockchain minus who tried the best to gain the data. There is much risk involved in the data related to healthcare management and can also harm the cost and all the activities regarding it as it is a very tedious process. The methods used these days for the security and privacy of the data are not adequate and sufficient. The privacy of the patient's medical data is essential these days as it can check the patient's condition. If privacy is not managed correctly, it can adversely affect stakeholders, minors, and patients. To avoid this, blockchain-based framework is being set up to complete security regarding the patient's information (Zhou et al., 2018).

7.3.15 SECURE MEDICAL DATA SHARING

The authors believed that there had been records in the electronic medical record with new technology. There is a case of database, which means information of the same patient is recorded in different hospitals. It can break the safety and security in the electronic medical record. These are not overcrowding and do not consume much energy. It helps to keep the record safe and secure. Health data management comprises the different patients who want their records to be secured in the blockchain. The record of a new patient is done in the same blockchain only. All the blockchains are connected and have some channels for their distribution. The connected blockchain has information about the previous block and also has a vast network. The advantage of making this system is that patients can later check their records, and it is easy to understand, can be distributed, secure, legal forms, and adequate. If any illegal method is practiced, it is shown in the record and then can be rectified. It identifies the type of data it shows to blockchain miners. It allows the entry to be done only by a few users. They can add information from different sources like hospital servers, physician offices, etc. It focuses on centralization (Fan et al., 2018).

7.3.16 LOCATION SHARING SCHEME

The authors thought that the place where patients are situated is a viewpoint when they keep mobile healthcare technologies. However, it faces a problem with protection and safety. This is the reason they have approved a multilevel scheme of blockchain-based location. It is adequate, real, and useful for implementing it in a real-life case. This scheme has played many roles and has its entity. It keeps the medical-related record safe and secure. It also keeps in check the user's information and corrects it in case it is wrong. Now comes the registration unit, which is responsible for providing the vital information about the users who want to do the entry in the system; after adding it once, they have to log in through the safe password and security while doing any transaction. A private accessible unit is a unit where two parties have involved that group together while exchanging through the proved channels. It works as a bridge between secure data and users saved in the blockchain (Ji et al., 2018).

7.4 CONCLUSION

It has been proved that blockchain has improved the healthcare system and motivated many people potentially and economically. The main focus is on managing the health record electronically through the blockchain system. It also allows us to take care of every segment that results in an exchange of the healthcare industry. Blockchain is shown as a paradigm changer by using its new idea for management, immutable audit trail, centralization, and robustness. It has been shown that applying the concept of blockchain not only improves the business but also helps to keep the record of the patient, scientist, and pharmaceutical industry. It also helps grow it through trustable trials, transparency, and primary focus on the research community. Adding the patient's consent regarding their treatment history and preferences on the blockchain will allow stakeholders to assess consent from any place and elevate the patient's care. There is a need for information blocking when anyone without the hospital's permission or the patient wants to see the patient's information. It also plays a vital role in building the quality and solving the issues related to sharing the data according to the given time. The paper has shown blockchain technology that has been remarkably done on medical healthcare by studying it properly. It also highlights the privacy and secrecy of the data related to the person's health.

CONFLICT OF INTEREST

None.

REFERENCES

Bartling, S. (2019). Blockchain for science and knowledge creation. In *Gesundheit Digital* (pp. 159–180). Berlin, Heidelberg: Springer.

Bartling, S., & Fecher, B. (2016). Blockchain for science and knowledge creation. doi: 10.5281/zenodo.60223.

Bates, M. (2018). Direct-to-consumer genetic testing: Is the public ready for simple, at-home DNA tests to detect disease risk? *IEEE Pulse, 9*(6), 11–14.

Benchoufi, M., Porcher, R., & Ravaud, P. (2017). Blockchain protocols in clinical trials: Transparency and traceability of consent. *F1000Research, 6,* 66.

Brandon, R. M., Podhorzer, M., & Pollak, T. H. (1991). Premiums without benefits: Waste and inefficiency in the commercial health insurance industry. *International Journal of Health Services: Planning, Administration, Evaluation, 21*(2), 265–283.

Cachin, C. (2016, July). Architecture of the hyperledger blockchain fabric. *In Workshop on Distributed Cryptocurrencies and Consensus Ledgers.* Zurich, Switzerland, (Vol. 310, No. 4).

Chan, A.-W., Tetzlaff, J. M., Altman, D. G., Dickersin, K., & Moher, D. (2013). SPIRIT 2013: New guidance for content of clinical trial protocols. *Lancet, 381*(9861), 91–92.

Colhoun, H. M., McKeigue, P. M., & Davey Smith, G. (2003). Problems of reporting genetic associations with complex outcomes. *Lancet, 361*(9360), 865–872.

CONSORT (2010). Retrieved December 17, 2020, from Consort-statement.org website: http://www.consort-statement.org/consort-2010.

Dai, H., Young, H. P., Durant, T. J. S., Gong, G., Kang, M., Krumholz, H. M., Jiang, L. (2018). TrialChain: A blockchain-based platform to validate data integrity in large, biomedical research studies. Retrieved from http://arxiv.org/abs/1807.03662.

Das, R. (2017, May 8). Does blockchain have a place in healthcare? *Forbes Magazine.* Retrieved from https://www.forbes.com/sites/reenitadas/2017/05/08/does-blockchain-have-a-place-in-healthcare/.

Daue, R. (2017, June 20). Falsified medicines. Retrieved December 18, 2020, from Europa.eu website: https://ec.europa.eu/health/human-use/falsified_medicines_en.

Dimitrov, D. V. (2016). Medical internet of things and big data in healthcare. *Healthcare Informatics Research, 22*(3), 156–163.

Downing, N. L., Adler-Milstein, J., Palma, J. P., Lane, S., Eisenberg, M., Sharp, C., Northern California HIE Collaborative. (2017). Health information exchange policies of 11 diverse health systems and the associated impact on volume of exchange. *Journal of the American Medical Informatics Association: JAMIA, 24*(1), 113–122.

Ekblaw, A., Azaria, A., Halamka, J. D., & Lippman, A. (2016). A case study for blockchain in healthcare: "MedRec" prototype for electronic health records and medical research data. *In Proceedings of IEEE Open & Big Data Conference.* Vienna, Austria, (Vol. 13, p. 13).

Ethereum Foundation. (2015). On public and private blockchains. Retrieved December 21, 2020, from Ethereum.org website: https://blog.ethereum.org/2015/08/07/on-public-and-private-blockchains/.

Fan, K., Wang, S., Ren, Y., Li, H., & Yang, Y. (2018). MedBlock: Efficient and secure medical data sharing via blockchain. *Journal of Medical Systems, 42*(8), 136.

Frankenfield, J. (2020, August 28). 51% attack. Retrieved December 5, 2020, from Investopedia.com website: https://www.investopedia.com/terms/1/51-attack.asp.

Genomes.io. (2020). Retrieved December 26, 2020, from Genomes.io website: https://genomes.io/blog/post/genomesio-for-rare-disease-research-9.

Gipp, B., Meuschke, N., & Gernandt, A. (2015). Decentralized trusted timestamping using the crypto currency Bitcoin. Retrieved from http://arxiv.org/abs/1502.04015.

Git. (2017). Retrieved December 17, 2020, from Git-scm.com website: https://git-scm.com/.

Gorman, L. (2006). The history of health care costs and health insurance. *Wisconsin Policy Research Institute Report, 19*(10), 1–31.

Graham, R. N. J., Perriss, R. W., & Scarsbrook, A. F. (2005). DICOM demystified: A review of digital file formats and their use in radiological practice. *Clinical Radiology, 60*(11), 1133–1140.

Griebel, L., Prokosch, H.-U., Köpcke, F., Toddenroth, D., Christoph, J., Leb, I., Sedlmayr, M. (2015). A scoping review of cloud computing in healthcare. *BMC Medical Informatics and Decision Making, 15*(1), 17.

Healthwizz. (2019). Virtual clinical trials: Changing perceptions. Retrieved December 26, 2020, from Healthwizz.com website: https://www.healthwizz.com/blog-posts-2/virtual-clinical-trials-changing-perceptions.

Hertig, A. (2018, June 8). Blockchain's once-feared 51% attack is now becoming regular: CoinDesk. Retrieved December 5, 2020, from CoinDesk website: https://www.coindesk.com/blockchains-feared-51-attack-now-becoming-regular.

Houston, M. S., Myers, J. D., Levens, S. P., McEvoy, M. T., Smith, S. A., Khandheria, B. K., Berry, D. J. (1999). Clinical consultations using store-and-forward telemedicine technology. *Mayo Clinic Proceedings, 74*(8), 764–769.

ICH E9 Expert Working Group. (1999). Statistical principles for clinical trials. *Statistics in Medicine, 18*, 1905–1942.

Idrees, S. M., Nowostawski, M., & Jameel, R. (2021). Blockchain-based digital contact tracing apps for COVID-19 pandemic management: Issues, challenges, solutions, and future directions. *JMIR Medical Informatics, 9*(2), e25245.

Idrees, S.M.; Nowostawski, M.; Jameel, R.; Mourya, A.K. Security Aspects of Blockchain Technology Intended for Industrial Applications. Electronics 2021, 10, 951. https://doi.org/10.3390/electronics10080951

Ioannidis, J. P. A. (2003). Genetic associations: False or true? *Trends in Molecular Medicine, 9*(4), 135–138.

Ioannidis, J. P. A. (2005). Why most published research findings are false. *PLoS Medicine, 2*(8), e124.

Ioannidis, J. P. A., Evans, S. J. W., Gøtzsche, P. C., O'Neill, R. T., Altman, D. G., Schulz, K., ... CONSORT Group. (2004). Better reporting of harms in randomized trials: An extension of the CONSORT statement. *Annals of Internal Medicine, 141*(10), 781–788.

Irving, G., & Holden, J. (2016). How blockchain-timestamped protocols could improve the trustworthiness of medical science. *F1000Research, 5*, 222.

Jayachandran, P. (2017, May 31). IBM Research. *The Difference Between Public and Private Blockchain.* Ibm.Com. https://www.ibm.com/blogs/blockchain/2017/05/the-difference-between-public-and-private-blockchain/

Ji, Y., Zhang, J., Ma, J., Yang, C., & Yao, X. (2018). BMPLS: Blockchain-based multi-level privacy-preserving location sharing scheme for telecare medical information systems. *Journal of Medical Systems, 42*(8), 147.

Kaye, J., Whitley, E. A., Lund, D., Morrison, M., Teare, H., & Melham, K. (2015). Dynamic consent: a patient interface for twenty-first century research networks. *European Journal of Human Genetics: EJHG, 23*(2), 141–146.

Ledger. (2019, October 23). What is blockchain? Retrieved December 4, 2020, from Ledger. com website: https://www.ledger.com/academy/blockchain/what-is-blockchain/.

Li, Z., Wu, H., King, B., Ben Miled, Z., Wassick, J., & Tazelaar, J. (2017). On the integration of event-based and transaction-based architectures for supply chains. *2017 IEEE 37th International Conference on Distributed Computing Systems Workshops (ICDCSW)*, IEEE, Atlanta, GA.

Li, H., Zhu, L., Shen, M., Gao, F., Tao, X., & Liu, S. (2018). Blockchain-based data preservation system for medical data. *Journal of Medical Systems, 42*(8), 141.

Linn, L. A., & Koo, M. B. (2020). Blockchain for health data and its potential use in health IT and health care related research. Retrieved December 5, 2020, from Truevaluemetrics. org website: http://www.truevaluemetrics.org/DBpdfs/Technology/Blockchain/11-74-ablockchainforhealthcare.pdf.

Lu, Q., & Xu, X. (2017). Adaptable blockchain-based systems: A case study for product traceability. *IEEE Software, 34*(6), 21–27.

Mandl, K. D. (2001). Public standards and patients' control: How to keep electronic medical records accessible but private commentary: Open approaches to electronic patient records Commentary: A patient's viewpoint. *BMJ (Clinical Research Ed.), 322*(7281), 283–287.

Марков, А. (2018, January 13). Способыприменениятехнологииблокчейн в медицине. Retrieved December 16, 2020, from Miningbitcoinguide.com website: https://miningbitcoinguide.com/technology/blokchejn-v-meditsine.

Mathieu, S., Boutron, I., Moher, D., Altman, D. G., & Ravaud, P. (2009). Comparison of registered and published primary outcomes in randomized controlled trials. *JAMA: The Journal of the American Medical Association, 302*(9), 977–984.

Mearian, L. (2019, September 23). How pharma will soon use blockchain to track your drugs. Retrieved December 17, 2020, from Computerworld.com website: https://www.computerworld.com/article/3439843/how-pharma-will-soon-use-blockchain-to-track-your-drugs.html.

Medicalchain. (2020, February 21). Is blockchain the answer to health record privacy concerns? Retrieved December 26, 2020, from Medicalchain.com website: https://medicalchain.com/en/is-blockchain-the-answer-to-health-record-privacy-concerns/.

Mettler, M. (2016). Blockchain technology in healthcare: The revolution starts here. *2016 IEEE 18th International Conference on E-Health Networking, Applications and Services (Healthcom)*, IEEE. Munich, Germany.

Moher, D., Cook, D. J., Eastwood, S., Olkin, I., Rennie, D., & Stroup, D. F. (1999). Improving the quality of reports of meta-analyses of randomised controlled trials: The QUOROM statement. *Lancet, 354*(9193), 1896–1900.

Moher, D., Dulberg, C. S., & Wells, G. A. (1994). Statistical power, sample size, and their reporting in randomized controlled trials. *JAMA: The Journal of the American Medical Association, 272*(2), 122–124.

Mulward, S., & Gotzsche, P. C. (1996). Sample size of randomized double-blind trials 1976–1991. *Danish Medical Bulletin, 43*(1), 96–98.

Collins, F.S. (2019, June 11). New collaboration and our vision for the future of genomics. Retrieved December 26, 2020, from Nebula.org website: https://blog.nebula.org/emdserono-collaboration/.

Omar, I., Jayaraman, R., Salah, K., Yaqoob, I., & Ellahham, S. (2020). Applications of blockchain technology in clinical trials: Review and open challenges. doi: 10.36227/techrxiv.12635783.v1.

Omenn, G. S., Nass, S. J., & Micheel, C. M. (Eds.). (2012). *Evolution of Translational Omics: Lessons Learned and the Path Forward*. Washington, DC: National Academies Press.

Perez-Marco, R. (2016). Bitcoin and decentralized trust protocols. Retrieved from http://arxiv.org/abs/1601.05254.

Peters, G. W., & Panayi, E. (2016). Understanding modern banking ledgers through block-chain technologies: Future of transaction processing and smart contracts on the Internet of money. In P. Tasca, L. Pelizzon, T. Aste, & N. Perony (Eds), *Banking Beyond Banks and Money* (pp. 239–278). Cham: Springer International Publishing.

Plotnikov, V., & Kuznetsova, V. (2018). The prospects for the use of digital technology "Blockchain" in the pharmaceutical market. *MATEC Web of Conferences,* Russia, *193*, 02029.

Salah, K., Rehman, M. H., Nizamuddin, N., & Al-Fuqaha, A. (2019). Blockchain for AI: Review and open research challenges. *IEEE Access: Practical Innovations, Open Solutions, 7*, 1–1.

Sandve, G. K., Nekrutenko, A., Taylor, J., & Hovig, E. (2013). Ten simple rules for reproducible computational research. *PLoS Computational Biology, 9*(10), e1003285.

Taylor, P. (2016, April 27). Applying blockchain technology to medicine traceability. Retrieved December 16, 2020, from Securingindustry.com website: https://www.securingindustry.com/pharmaceuticals/applying-blockchain-technology-to-medicine-traceability/s40/a2766/.

Singh, N. (2019, January 21). Blockchain for healthcare: Use cases and applications. Retrieved December 4, 2020, from 101 Blockchains.com website: https://101blockchains.com/blockchain-for-healthcare/.

Sylim, P., Liu, F., Marcelo, A., & Fontelo, P. (2018). Blockchain technology for detecting falsified and substandard drugs in distribution: Pharmaceutical supply chain intervention. *JMIR Research Protocols, 7*(9), e10163.

Tian, F. (2017). A supply chain traceability system for food safety based on HACCP, block-chain & Internet of things. *2017 International Conference on Service Systems and Service Management,* IEEE, Dalian, China.

Toyoda, K., Mathiopoulos, P. T., Sasase, I., & Ohtsuki, T. (2017). A novel blockchain-based product ownership management system (POMS) for anti-counterfeits in the post supply chain. *IEEE Access: Practical Innovations, Open Solutions, 5*, 17465–17477.

Trujllo, G., & Guillermo, C. (2018). The role of blockchain in the pharmaceutical industry supply chain as a tool for reducing the flow of counterfeit drugs (Doctoral dissertation, Ph. D. Thesis, Dublin Business School, Dublin, Ireland).

Vahdati, M., GholizadehHamlAbadi, K., & Saghiri, A. M. (2021). IoT-based healthcare monitoring using blockchain. In *Studies in Big Data* (pp. 141–170). Singapore: *Springer.*

WHO | WHO Data Set. (2020). Retrieved from https://www.who.int/ictrp/network/trds/en/.

Wisniewska, A. (2016). *Altcoins.* Institute of Economic Research.

Yang, H., & B Yang, B. (2018). A blockchain -based approach to the secure sharing of healthcare data. In A. J. Laszlo Erdodi (Ed.), *Norsk Informasjonssikkerhetskonferanse 2017* (pp. 100–111). Nisk Journal.

Zajc, T. (2018, October 29). F020 Blockchain, value of data, and the role of legislation with adoption (Ray Dogum, Health Unchained). Retrieved December 26, 2020, from Faces Of Digital Health website: https://medium.com/faces-of-digital-health/f020-blockchain-value-of-data-and-the-role-of-legislation-with-adoption-ray-dogum-health-80919d909e97.

Zheng, Z., Xie, S., Dai, H., Chen, X., & Wang, H. (2017). An overview of blockchain technology: Architecture, consensus, and future trends. *2017 IEEE International Congress on Big Data (BigData Congress)*, IEEE.

Zhou, L., Wang, L., & Sun, Y. (2018). MIStore: A blockchain-based medical insurance storage system. *Journal of Medical Systems, 42*(8), 149.

8 Computing Techniques for Securing Healthcare Data with Blockchain Technology

Apurva Saxena Verma
Researcher Computer science

Anubha Dubey
Independent researcher and analyst

CONTENTS

DOI: 10.1201/9781003141471-8

8.1   INTRODUCTION

Cloud computing has been valuable to many IT environments due to its competence and accessibility. Moreover, cloud security and privacy concerns have been discussed in terms of significant security elements: confidentiality, integrity, access control, authentication, and so on. If the client data is disclosed in the cloud computing environment, financial and psychological compensations can occur due to the leak of users' sensitive information. The security of the data, such as confidentiality and integrity, in the cloud computing environment, is mainly. Its services Data as a Service (DAAS), Software as a Service (SAAS), Platform as a Service (PAAS), and Infrastructure as a Service (IAAS) allow users to protect data at each level. These services are better enough for storing and analyzing patient's data in a secure manner. To develop a secure environment, any of these services are used in public or private cloud. Sometimes, hybrid clouds are also used for data storage and security as per the requirement of the industry (healthcare also).

8.1.1   BLOCKCHAIN IN CLOUD

Blockchain is a representative technology for ensuring secrecy suggested by Dejan V. et al. (2018). If combined with the cloud computing environment, blockchain can be promoted to a suitable service that provides stronger security. User secrecy can be ensured if the blockchain method is used when saving the client information in the cloud computing environment.

Blockchain technology is a center of improvement that is built about the perception of a circulated agreement ledger. Here the ledger is reserved and sustained on a scattered system of computers said by Seyednima, K. (2019). This given ledger creates it probable for the whole network to mutually create, evolve, and keep follow of single undeniable record of transactions, and it is nowadays mainly recognized as the blockchain. This most important expertise purpose has been a crypto currency known as Bitcoin. It is said to be a ledger popularly known as the blockchain, through which it got its first name suggested by Zhou, Y. (2018).

It is a worldwide circulated ledger, which supports the association of resources crosswise the globe in moments, with the least transaction charge. These resources can be signified digitally. Blockchain technology is recognized as a distributed ledger technology for peer-to-peer (P2P) network data transactions digitally that might be circulated publicly or privately to all users (Idrees et. al., 2021). This way allows data to be stored in a reliable and provable form as told by Seyednima, K. (2019). A further main concept of this technology is the smart deal, an authorized necessary rule that consists of a customizable set of laws below which different groups agree to interact with each other. This technology has several smart deal applications in several areas, such as energy resources, financial services, and healthcare. This technology proposes precision and eliminates the requirement for third-party mediators. It uses consent mechanisms and cryptography to validate the authority of a transaction in a trustless environment.

8.1.2. BACKGROUND

Some of the interesting papers are discussed below to understand the blockchain technology process. The author (Chukwu, E., Garg, L. 2020) tried to explain blockchain which is capable of between others to deal with the various EHR dares, mainly information along with stakeholder. Numerous blockchain-in-healthcare structures were planned; a few prototyped get executed. In this paper, methodological and architectural study of some 61 editorials for privacy, security, cost, and performance was completed in detail. According to this study, blockchain was created to resolve the trust, security, and privacy limitations of conventional EHRs.

Here in this author (Fran, C., 2018) work provides an organized review of blockchain-based applications crossways multiple areas. The researcher's plan is to study the present state of blockchain technology and its purposes and to emphasize specific characteristics of this technology that can revolutionize practices (Gendal.2015).

The author (Julija, G., Andrejs, R. 2018) describes Blockchain technology as well as its merits and demerits. Several executed applications of blockchain skills are considered. This paper wants to explore services and difficulties associated with blockchain integration. The purpose of study from the author (Anton, H., 2019) was to thoroughly assess, evaluate and combine peer-reviewed periodical proposing to use blockchain to recover processes and services in the healthcare organization.

This work of the author (Tanesh, K., 2018) shows the challenges and problems desired to tenacity previous to the victorious acceptance of blockchain technology in healthcare organizations. Moreover, the author (Jun, L., 2020) introduces the smart bond for blockchain-based healthcare systems that are essential for pre-defined contracts. According to this, the blockchain is used to handle and coordinate the namespace and execute an index for content metadata in organizing to maintain content distribution and purchase. As per Ho, P. (2017), blockchain can be useful beyond the Internet of Things (IoT) background. Its functions are estimated to develop. Cloud computing also has been noticeably adopted in the new era of technology environments for its competence and accessibility. Here they discuss the perception of blockchain technology and its research developments.

8.1.3 GLIMPSES OF MACHINE LEARNING

Machine learning (ML) is best known for its experience-based applications which will develop different models for patterns identified. ML is a scientific discipline that got the term from Arthur Samuel (Vapnik, V. 1995).It is a technology that teaches computers how to use different algorithms without being precisely programmed. It's a diverse field combination like philosophy, statistics, control theory, psychology, and artificial intelligence. Large databases in hospital records contain different patterns that can be discovered simultaneously for particular disease diagnosis and treatment (Srinivas, K., 2020; Dubey A., 2018). ML models basically work on patterns identified by computer programming or algorithms.

8.1.4 MACHINE LEARNING AND BLOCKCHAIN CHNOLOGY

These technologies with blockchain make the system smarter and easy to work with. ML can also help in the security of electronic patient data. The EMR (electronic medical record) is needed to be protected from business or hackers. During data sharing, hacking can be done. Therefore, in our study, we developed a proposed model for blockchain. All the data sharing routes should be in monitoring in the cloud environment. The data can be collected from patient's self-information, doctor visit, doctor suggested medicines, or different blood tests. All these data generated sources are very important to be saved from malicious activity. These data need to be analyzed further for treatment enhancement of some critical patients. They are helpful in predictions for further diagnosis based on symptoms. Different IoT is linked purposefully to store and save data in a network based on the cloud. The blockchain is integrated with this cloud network works better for EMR data security.

On the basis of data, different databases are formed which are linked together. This will reduce time, errors like duplication, missing values, entry correction, etc. Blockchain will focus on the data and eliminating data-related issues. These ML models are based on chain segments in the entire data set. Hence mistakes are avoided by the system.

8.1.5 MACHINE LEARNING APPLICATION IN THE BLOCKCHAIN NETWORK

Persons can generate fake identity but our proposed system ML-based blockchain network will control all types of consensus as explained by Julija, G., Andrejs, R. 2018). Here ML plays a powerful role in identifying signature patterns for any kind of fraud. This model can be effective in data traffic too. An efficient and effective ML algorithm is used to analyze the traffic in data in the blockchain network. This is well designed to work securely in the cloud environment as Blockchain as a Service (BAAS). ML models work well with input data, and by the statistical analysis which is inbuilt, there is a system that makes a prediction and gives the updated output. This analysis helps to create a decision process for doctors and stakeholders. In the case of COVID-19, according to the symptoms identified, ML models help to diagnose the disease at low, medium, and high levels, and treatment will be decided by the healthcare providers. This ML model works in real time. This is very important for patients and doctors. In this chapter, we are discussing how ML models work well in a blockchain network. These models are helping in observing COVID patient's everyday behavior of medicine suitability or side reactions. This is the basic part of the study to understand the disease like COVID-19. Data of all the severe patients are stored in a network that is monitored by a cloud (as shown in Figure 8.1).

The ML algorithm is of four types: supervised, semisupervised, unsupervised, and reinforcement learning. In our study, we used supervised ML models, and these use statistical models to predict to know the predicted desired output which classifies the correct label (Srinivas, K., 2020). Basically, a decision tree is used in the classification and prediction of diseases (Dubey A. 2010) and treatment (Dubey A., 2018).

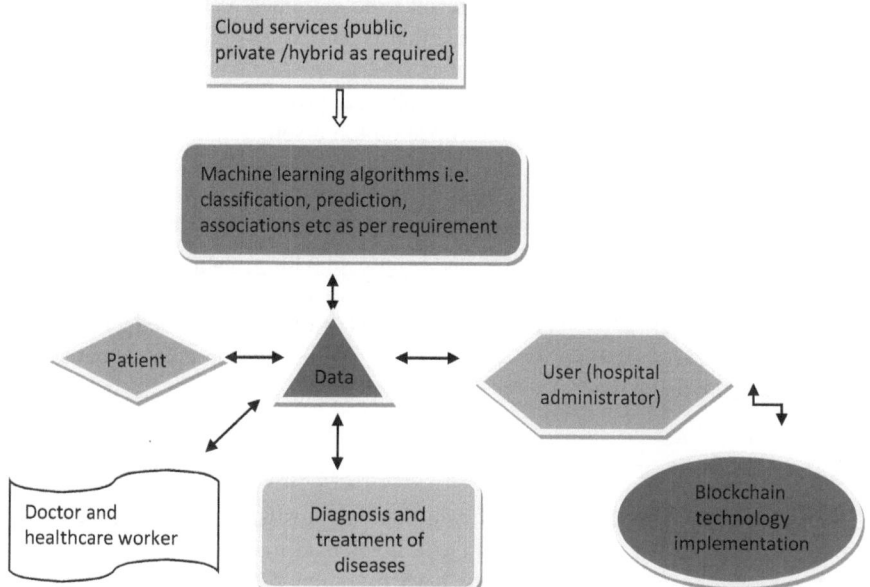

FIGURE 8.1 Architecture of ML in healthcare.

8.2 BLOCKCHAIN

It is a mainly gifted and innovatory technology. It helps to cut down risk, strikeout scam, and take intelligibility in a scalable method in numerous uses. The blockchain has been depicted as "an unwrap, distributed ledger that can trace connections among two parties proficiently, in a provable and stable way". This technology blockchain contains of three important concepts: blocks, nodes, and miners.

8.2.1 Core Components of Blockchain: The Components of Blockchain Are Described As

[a] **Blocks** : Each sequence contains many blocks, and each block has three vital essentials. The block contains data.
  • A nonce contains 32-bit whole number. The nonce is arbitrarily produced at the time of block is formed, which then produced header hash of a block.
  • This has his linked to the nonce has 256-bit number. It starts with zeroes. The first block of a series is formed; a nonce produced the cryptographic hash through (Gendal, 2015). The data in the block is measured marked and perpetually attached to the nonce and hash except it is extracted.
[b] **Miners:** They produce new blocks on the sequence through a method known mining. In a blockchain, each block kept its possessed exclusive nonce. Here hash mentions the prior block in the sequence, thus drawing out a block is tough (Gendal, 2015).

They use unique software to resolve the extremely complex mathematics difficulty of discovering a nonce that creates an established hash. When that hash gets generated, then miners said as "golden nonce" and the block further appended to the sequence. A block is productively mined, and this amendment is accepted by every node on the given system of network and miner pleased monetarily.

[c] **Nodes:** Here concept used in blockchain technology is decentralization. A distributed ledger contains the nodes attached in sequence (Gendal, 2015). All nodes have their copy of the blockchain, and the system agrees algorithmically for any new block in the sequence to get simplified, reliance, and confirmed. While blockchain is translucent, each act in the ledger can be naturally checked. Effectively, blockchain can be considered as scalable of trust using technology.

8.2.2 WORKING OF A BLOCKCHAIN

In blockchain, each block consists of data that can be shared across the network to a particular block of a person. Every block holds data, hash function of the earlier block, its own hash function, the next hash function of the connected block, and transaction details as shown in Figure 8.2. Here blockchain works in five stages as follows as defined by Zhou, Y., 2018):

- Description of transaction
- Verification of transaction
- Construction of block
- Validation of block
- Block attaching
    (i) **Description of Transaction**: Here the sender of the block forms a transaction and broadcast in the group. The broadcast note includes particulars of the public address of receiver, rate of the hash function, and a cryptographic digitally signature that confirms the validity of the transaction.

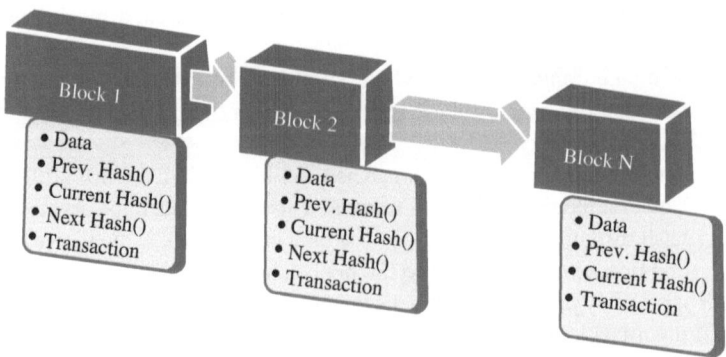

FIGURE 8.2 An overview of blockchain.

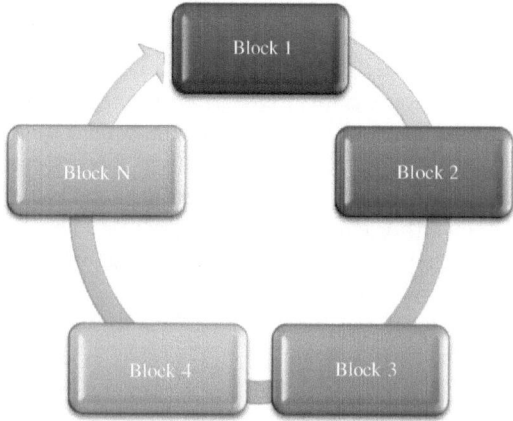

FIGURE 8.3 Blockchain network.

(ii) **Verification of Transaction**: A note is accepted by the system of the nodes (users), and they validate the legality of the note by decrypting it through the digital signature. A transaction is genuine when it is placed to a concern block in a network as shown in Figure 8.3.

(iii) **Construction of Block**: All transactions get placed collectively in a reorganized edition of the ledger, said to a block, in the system of network. At a precise time period, the particular node transmits in the block in the system of network for confirmation.

(iv) **Validation of Block**: Validated nodes in the system of the network accept the planned block and make effort to confirm it throughout in a repeated process that involves consent from the entire network. Various kind of blockchain has networks and uses different kinds of confirmation techniques. Bitcoin in blockchain applies a practice known to be a "proof-of-work". Ripple applies "Circulated Consensus". Ethereum applies "proof-of-stake". These different practices have various merits and demerits. A common point to ensure that each transaction is legal and creates counterfeit which is not viable.

(v) **Validation of Block:** When all the transactions are authenticated, the original block is "chained" into the method said to be a blockchain. This new existing state of the ledger gets transmitted in the system of the network. Entire process gets accomplished in few seconds.

8.2.3 BLOCKCHAIN CLASSES

Blockchain is divided into two classes: public chain (Permission less) and consortium or private chain (Permission) (Gendal, 2015).

- **Public Chain (Permission Less Ledger):** The public chain is symbolized by Bitcoin and Ethereum. Everyone can be part of it, and all proceedings are available in the public. In permission-less ledgers, it's allowing the process to join into the connections scheme. A replica of the blockchain ledger can be downloaded by anyone and capable to connect as mysterious, thorough proof-of-work (Jun L. 2020).

- **Consortium or Private Chain (Permission Ledger):** Consortium chains consist of a number of blockchain agreements formed by a definite group of people. Similarly, the transaction proceedings are reserved in the blockchain, but they are only accessible by consortium members. A pre-selected set of nodes is done through the validation process. The right to use read mode in the blockchain is restricted to a specific figure of applicants, such as auditors allowed by government (Qiu, C., 2018).
- Neither free nor as large as a public chain. This kind of blockchain is best characterized by the hyperledger.

8.3 HEALTHCARE SECTOR USED BLOCKCHAIN TECHNOLOGY

Figure 8.4 explains that healthcare systems like hospital and research lab are connected to the digital system in the cloud environment, which provides security to the data stored in it. Here in the pandemic time, information of the patients who are suffering from different diseases and those are affected by COVID get stored in the electronic system. Detail history of every patient with their corresponding doctor is stored in the database which is secured in the cloud environment which is monitored constantly. The hospital research laboratory is also connected and secured in different ways in the cloud by administrators and lab workers who are only able to login. The supply chain of all the medical types of equipment and other items information is get stored in the central database. Insurance claims related to the treatments are all stored in the related patient's database. All these treatments and their payments are done electronically which is secured under a blockchain network.

8.3.1 Components of Digital Health System

(i) **Digital Store Health Database:** In many cases, data is not secured due to which high-quality data get hacked or being misused from attacker. In this, digitized environment ML is used in the cloud environment across a network for healthcare organizations using blockchain. Therefore, union of all of the data across the network gets maximum benefits. Blockchain can be used to place metadata, pointers, and hash codes about data that currently in the network within various healthcare organizations contributing to a blockchain network. Further healthcare organizations sharing this network can use this information on the blockchain to explore, determine, trace, and consequently securely recover data from peers as essential to build the ML model. Blockchain can be used to follow the origin, accuracy, and reliability of data.

(ii) **Insurance Company:** Here blockchain permits the following data sets to assemble and instruct through ML models. If the origin of data is followed on the blockchain, then this information can be taken into deliberation in sorting out the highest quality data as company guidelines and tie-up have been described in detail and must be secure. Through ML, it is essential

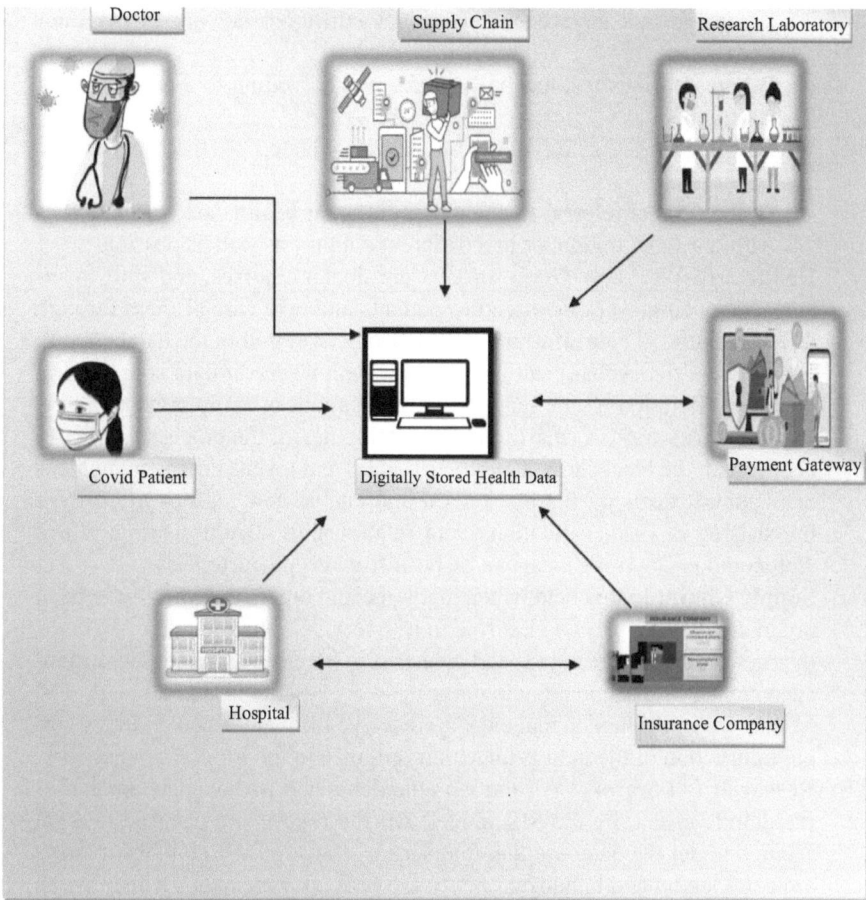

FIGURE 8.4 Components of digitally stored data in healthcare virtual system.

to protect their integrity and be able to confirm their faithfulness using a blockchain network. ML can be shared using blockchain, and more swiftly develop and grown through partnership across a network of healthcare organizations working independently.

(iii) **Patients:** Patients are in need of privacy which is the most important entity to engage and build trust with ML as they are the source of data. Blockchain allows a level of patient commitment that allows them to evaluate their records, modify as needed, and approve (opt-in/opt-out) to their participation. This is still more important going further where masses of the patient data will come from "consumer health care center". Through this security, patient's data will always secure and get checked through ML at each stage of verification as follows:

- Differentiate among patients from non-COVID to COVID patients at the time of registration.

- When patients have been referring to different doctors as per their treatments.
- Patients various test has been performed according to their history of treatments.
- Insurance claims are done by patients related to their prescribed treatment.
- At the time of referral to one patient to other health care organizations within a state, region, or in a different country as well as possible.

(iv) **Healthcare Workers:** These workers are doctors, nurses, and staff members. Many employees do attend to patients and take care of them through different duties. Their information has also been stored in the databases. In this network, blockchain can provide precision wherever data comes from; a model is built to provide security and validations of assumption results.

(v) **Payment Gateway:** A smart treaty can computerize the processing of connections on the blockchain. Cryptocurrencies and tokens are the main ideas of the smart deals on the blockchain and enable new reasons to catalyze the sharing of data, validations, and relationships. DAOs (Decentralized Autonomous Organizations) can be built from cryptocurrencies.

(vi) **Supply Chain:** In this field, when medicine and other equipment have been ordered, database plays a vital role in it. Every information related to items that get ordered, exchanged, and returned is precisely defined. Here management works day and night to make the work systematic and efficient. The ML model works here to make the system free from any attacker. Every single transaction of the item is under surveillance in the Blockchain network.

(vii) **Research Laboratory:** All the lab attendants and pathologists are authorized and verified by the ML model. All the reports are checked and get secured under the database that manages by the administrator. Test reports are confidential and handover only to the patients which are verified by the authenticate process done under the ML model. This model works in the blockchain network under the continuous monitoring of the cloud platform.

(viii) **Healthcare Organization:**Each healthcare organization constructs this experience separately and redundantly then it will take a long time. Here blockchain is used to allow sharing of ML model assumption results and validations of those results across a network of healthcare organizations. Trust builds rapidly,progresses,and decreases costs. If the organization is ever in need to audit an assumption result,as part of a regular validation,then blockchain can offer a complete audit trail (Morgen, P., 2017).

According to (Wasim, 2018),ML-based architecture is used to monitor contract breaches. He used an unsupervised ML algorithm called the probability-based factor model to issue injunctions (Wang, 2018). This model simulated using three service providers Redis (Redis, 2019), MongoDB (Mongo DB accessed, 2019), and Memcached Servers (Memacached servers accessed, 2019). The more the services occupied,the more complex operation is likely to perform.

8.4 BLOCKCHAIN IN BIG DATA ERA

This is the data-generated era. Everywhere huge data is collected. In our proposed system, all the generated data is used well,stored,and secured. It is linked with IoT,smartphones,and other computing devices (Qiu, C. 2018; Bhatia, J. 2019),. All electronic medical data is highly valuable. As ML is implemented,all kind of electronic health data is used and classified as per need, and predictions can be made about any disease outcome,patient's recovery,etc. In this COVID time,contactless work is appreciated. Hence our model or system works well in the COVID case. According to the need,ML models work in a supervised, semi-supervised, or reinforcement way (Velankar, 2018). This will help in any hidden patterns that need to be studied is considered. Now the society needs these models-based blockchain network. Further bitcoin mining is also introduced with an artificial neural network to remove the irrelevant data.It is used in a state evolution algorithm that is based on hash value,nonce,address,and transaction data in a blockchain network.

8.5 BLOCKCHAIN IN REAL TIME DATA

All kinds of electronic data are enablingreal-time analytics whether it is accessible, transactional, and operational Liu, C., (2015). It is using in-memory computing in blockchain-based cloud environment which is monitored, and data is widely updated. Every time analytics accuracy is improved, and the predictive behaviors of ML models are achieved. Blockchain-based network makes secure payment Liu, C., (2015). This blockchain hinders the cross geographic hindrances;the framework of ML and blockchain accomplishes the goal of data analysis and storage in secure cloud environment. This makes fast business, and all suspicious activities are recorded.According to (Qiu, C. 2018; Bhatia, J. 2019), the performance level of the software-defined vehicular network is improved using Q-learning method,and SDVN based on real-time city traffic study in vehicular ad hoc networkenvironment (VANETs) (Qiu, C. 2018; Bhatia, J. 2019),. Liu, C., (2015) proposed a data collection framework for Industrial–IoT applications (IIOT) with the combination of deep reinforcement learning and ethereum blockchain which can be implemented in healthcare sector Liu, C., (2015).

8.6 OUR PROPOSED WORK

In Figure 8.5, our proposed SeMB (Security-enhanced Machine learning Blockchain) model is designed in the cloud environment which is constantly monitored by the server and gets secured by any malicious attacker. Here in the cloud environment MFA (Multi-Factor Authentication) security is used to enter strongly in the blockchain implemented environment. Access permits by those having the authority to enter the cloud scenario.Here blockchain technology is implemented where every person has his own block in this blockchain network under a cloud platform. The first level is to enter into the network through the login credential which is unique and given to every

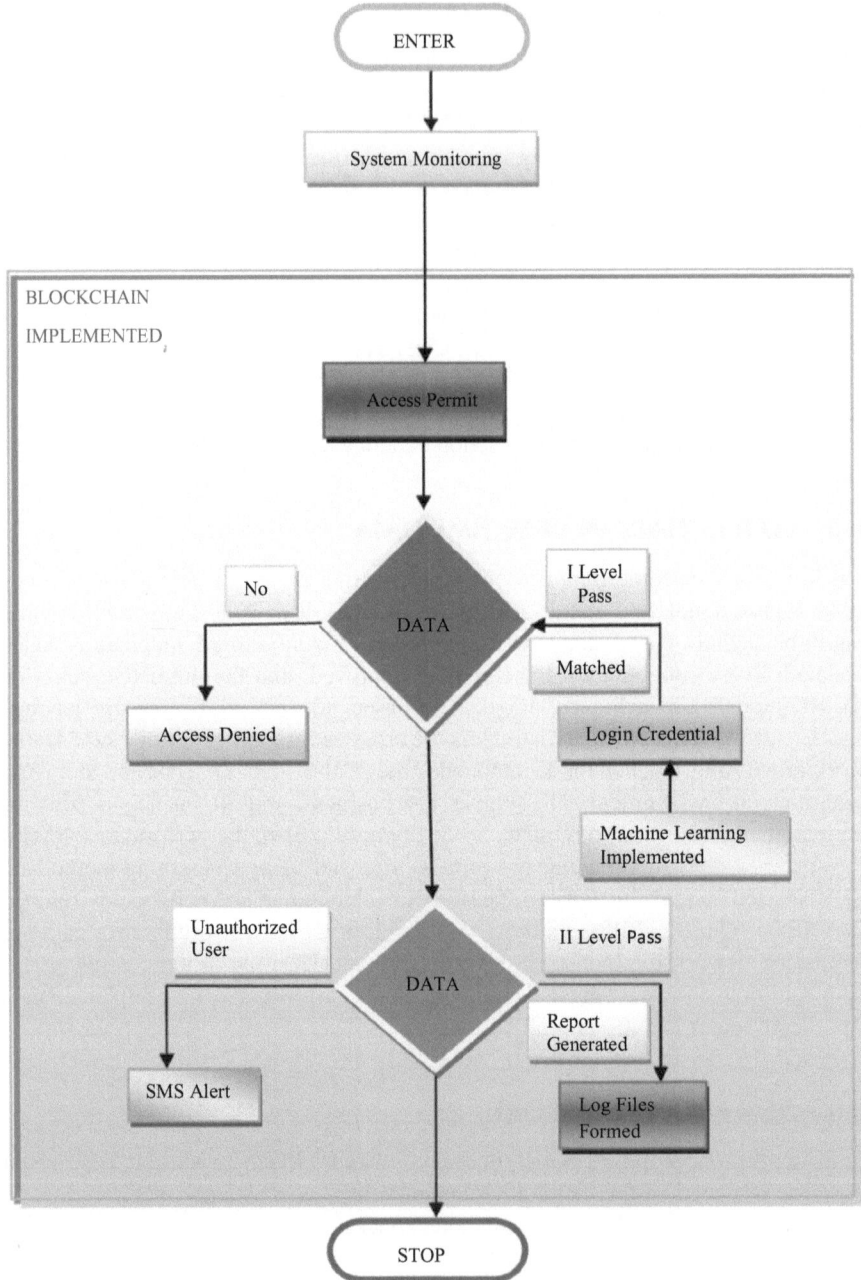

FIGURE 8.5 Flowchart of a SeMB (Security-enhanced Machine learning Blockchain) model.

block in the blockchain network. If any new person tries to enter into this network whose block has not created,it's assumed to be an unauthorized person and access will be denied. In the second level, every data which is stored gets secured; in the network, incoming and outgoing traffic will be monitored and logfiles generated. If some malicious acts happen the alert is generated through an alarm at the server site.

Steps to be followed in Security enhancement Machine Learning Blockchain (SeMB) model:

1. Any user needs to be authenticating by the blockchain system.
2. In cloud network,blockchain provides high security and is trustworthy.
3. The ML models are integrated with blockchain are sustainable.
4. Blockchain helps in incentive-based system.
5. The more the medical data available,ML model behaves more accurately.
6. All the computations are worked simultaneously with ML models.
7. In blockchain payment, process is also secure.
8. Mostly operated blockchain toolisEthereum,which is used for decentralized machines in one hospital.
9. As per requirement, this tool can be used to connect other machines in the world in a blockchain-based cloud network.

In this, the authors tried to include all the aspects which are required for the success of a model in the healthcare industry. As we all know this is the shining industry day by day. All are connected one in one at any period of time during life. So it is very essential that this sector would be one of the safest and secure where patients can rely upon. Kept this in mind,we authors take the opportunity to propose or build a system in the name of the SeMB model. The functionality of SeMB models is:

(i) **Preventing:** In our proposed SeMB model, we try to prevent the attacker to enter into the network from the entrylevel into any cloud environment such as AWS, Azure, OCP (Oracle Cloud Provider),GCP(Google Cloud Provider),IBM. At the time of login in second level inside the blockchain network with the use of ML algorithm no malicious activity can be possible.

(ii) **Predicting:** Here in this stage at the first level in blockchain network technology in our model at the time of login if the attacker wants to enter access will be denied. If some tries to modify the data log files formed and the report generated. Alert will be there at the server site through SMS. Here machine learning algorithms are also worked to classify disease in its stage as data is provided. Like COVID data,it is identified in which stage low,medium, and high. So the prediction of disease could be possible.

(iii) **Monitoring:** In our model at this stage, monitoring will be continuous of the whole network in the cloud environment. There are many cloud service provider which can provide these kinds of services for the security purpose. ML models help to monitor the treatment process and medications.

(iv) **Detection:** At the stage of the ML algorithm in our model at the login time,it can detect the user in various forms to detect the validation. In a blockchain,network security is present at all the nodes of a block so that malicious activity can be detected and stop at that level.

(v) **Blockchain Response:** Here response of blockchain in our SeMB model is to provide top security at each level of it. Implementation of blockchain in our network gives the support to our data get secure through the blocks which are get connected and shared. Everyone's information of one block will be shared by each of the blocks in the network. An attacker cannot harm anyone's data as it gets informed by everyone present in the network.

8.6.2 APPLICATIONS

The partnership of blockchain with ML techniques leaves no point left to make healthcare system data safe and secure. These revolutionizing technologies provide doctors the opportunity to provide better treatment to patients' satisfaction. The smart devices are there to interact with healthcare providers for proper patient behavior each and every time and making ML models successful. ML makes patient service quick, efficient, and automated to fulfill all the needs. An automL model is also proposed by Wang (2018), which can be implemented in blockchain-derived applications.

This ledger technology assists the secure transfer of patient medical records, directs the medicine supply chain, and helps healthcare researchers unlock genetic code explained by author (Chukwu, E., Garg, L., 2020).

- Blockchain is by now being used to do the lot for securely encrypts patient data to control the occurrence of detrimental diseases defined by Fran, C. (2018).Estonia is one of the countries which implemented blockchain in the healthcare system (Chawathe, S. 2018).
- All the country's healthcare invoice is handled on a blockchain, 95% of health information is ledger-based and 99% of all treatment information is digital suggested by Anton, H. (2019).
- The prospect of genomics to recover the expectations of human health. Blockchain is an ideal fit for this increasing business as it can carefully house billions of genetic facts (Fedorov, A.K., 2018).

8.6.3 ADVANTAGES AND DISADVANTAGES OF BLOCKCHAIN

All the developed techniques have their own pros and cons. Some of the pros and cons are identified by us that are discussed below:

Advantages: This technology works on decentralized system (Julija, G., Andrejs, R., 2018).

- An each act is traced in the blockchain, and records of data are accessible to the entire applicantin the system of blockchain which cannot remove. An outcome of the footage gives blockchain precision, incontrovertible, and reliability (Idrees, S.M., 2021).

- It is genuine and not useless communication among the mysterious people defined by author (Julija, G., Andrejs, R., 2018). The belief can amplify more as there can it contain extra mutual methods and reports.
- This unchallengeable attained on the connections which get approved and common crossways in this technology. The intelligibility of the blockchain is achieved on every connection; and it is copied to computer in this network explained by Julija, G., Andrejs, R., 2018).
  - The blockchain aims at the method by which it shows any troubles and approved them. This benefit creates this blockchain technology traceable (Idrees, S.M., 2021).
  - Blockchain technology is a trust worthy series of this cryptographic hash Julija, G., Andrejs, R., 2018). Every being that enters the blockchain is offered an exceptional identifier that associated with his account. The security in the blockchain is attained on the single entity access into the given system.

Disadvantages: The chief demerit of this technology is its elevated energy utilization. This is desirable for trusting a real-time ledger explained by Julija, G., Andrejs, R. (2018).

- An autograph or signature authentication is the major risk of the blockchain since every transaction should get signed through the cryptographic format, and the giant calculating authority is essential in working out the process to get signed.
- The next problem of this technology is to separate the series. The nodes that work on the earlier software will not allow entertaining in the latest connections (Fedorov, A.K., 2018).
- This soft fork creates an original rule set to implement in the blocks which present in the procedure. All nodes are reorganized to execute rules of the soft fork (Dejan, V., 2018).
- In the hard fork, loose the ruleset of the blocks in the procedure. Procedure is the identical in the soft fork process also, but merits and results are conflicting.
- Blockchain has developed at the time when new blocks associate with the series and the necessities of computing get increases (Idrees, S.M., 2021). All nodes cannot offer the essential capacity.

8.6.4 Issues and Challenges

As we worked on a ML-based blockchain system, issues and challenges are observed (Idrees, S.M., 2021). Some of them are discussed below:

a. **Is Blockchain Suitable?** Yes, blockchain is simple and applied to healthcare data and when the untrusted source of data is used, blockchain technology is applied (Salah, K., 2019).
b. **How Is the Blockchain Architecture?** The framework of blockchain-based ML must include network administration, hardware for mining

data, centered storage system, and best protocols for communication (Velankar, 2018).

c. **Is Data Secret?** This is quite challenging, as data is stored in a blockchain that is available to all the blockchain nodes (Chawathe, S., 2018). For data confidentiality, private blockchains are used for COVID and HIV like cases. This must be controlled access and end-to-end encrypted. Here ML models play a good role in imposing the barrier to limit the data. And the cloud environment is provided to secure all kinds of data (Dejan, V., 2018). As cloud computing monitors every time the data and when any malicious activity is tried to happen, the system generates an alarm or any signal to alert the administrator (Chawathe, S., 2018).

d. **What about the Computer or Virtual Memory of the System?** The size of blockchain keeps on growing day by day, and new blocks are added simultaneously. This will lead to the problem of system memory (Dejan, V., 2018). The performance of the system gets affected by these additions. That is a big problem as blockchain is inflexible. It can be sorted by applying ML algorithms that could sort irrelevant data and manage the computer or virtual memory (Fedorov, A.K., 2018).

8.7   CONCLUSION

Blockchain and ML are growing technologies and are in infancy. They are much more than studied and applied. In cloud networks, they work better, hence their capability is enriched day by day. Researchers around the world are working thoroughly to make our healthcare sector secure. SeMB model is developed for securing healthcare data. AutoML can be applied as more data and various ML algorithms are required in the specific section. Here discussed the advantages and disadvantages and also given solutions to issues identified during the development of the framework of the SeMB model. Future prospects of the work can be enhanced as follows:

(i) **Device Personalization**: When the quality of services is improved, personal wearable devices can also work accordingly (Fedorov, A.K., 2018). In the case of COVID, a health monitoring system can work very effectively in a smart way. The framework will provide smart decisions for COVID patients also to understand the COVID treatment process. Whenever any patient act as a user, a log is then generated with user data. This will help to recognize his whole old data like doctor prescription, blood test reports, etc. And this device generates alerts for the next visit to a doctor or any important test which is essential for patients.

(ii) **Quantum Supremacy**: Blockchain can be broken by quantum computers, as it is a very prominent technology. This is possible due to the hashing algorithm where the blockchain is used. It is used on a one-way function for encryption. Hence blockchain is a good digital storage framework. But favorably, quantum computing offers good luck to boost the performance of the blockchain as a quantum security system and cannot allow users to mimic another user. It is in an infancy stage and researchers are working on this, soon a system is developed that contains blockchain which provides security with quantum supremacy (Fedorov, A.K., 2018).

8.8 CONTRIBUTION

This chapter discusses the framework of SeMB model in which preventing and predicting through ML. In cloud monitoring, detecting works and responses generated through blockchain. This method is also helpful in storing healthcare data.

REFERENCES

Anton, H., Kralevskab, K., Gligoroskib, D., Pedersenc, S.A., Faxvaag, A. 2019. *Blockchain in healthcare and health sciences: A scoping review International. Journal of Medical Informatics*, 134, 104040. Published by Elsevier B.V., Available online: journal homepage: www.elsevier.com/locate/ijmedinf.

Bhatia, J., Dave, R., Bhayani, H., Tanwar, S., Nayyar, A. 2019. SDN-based real-time urban traffic analysis in vanet environment. *Computer Communications*, 149, 162–175.

Chawathe, S. 2018. Monitoring blockchains with self-organizing maps, In Proceedings of 17th IEEE International Conference on Trust, Security and Privacy in Computing and Communications/12th IEEE International Conference on Big Data Science and Engineering *(TrustCom/BigDataSE)*, New York, USA pp. 1870–1875.

Chukwu, E., Garg, L. 2020. A systematic review of blockchain in healthcare: Frameworks, prototypes, and implementations. *IEEE Access Date of Current Version*, 8, Liverpool, U.K. 21196–21214.

Dejan, V., Dijana, J., Siniša, R. 2018. Blockchain technology, bitcoin, and ethereum: A brief overview. *17th International Symposium Infoteh-Jahorina*, 21–23 March, 2018 East Sarajevo, Bosnia and Herzegovina.

Dubey, A. 2018. Biophotonics & machine learning model for the diagnosis AND treatment of HIV. *Bioscience Biotechnology Research Communications*, 11(1), 5–10.

Dubey, A., Pant, B., Adlakha, N. 2010. SVM model for amino acid composition based classification of HIV-1 groups, Bioinformatics and Biomedical Technology (ICBBT),*2010 International Conference*, IEEE Chengdu, China. doi: 10.1109/ICBBT.2010.5478996.

Fedorov, A.K., Kiktenko, E.O., Lvovsky, A.I. 2018. Quantum computers put blockchain security at risk. *Nature*, 563, 465–467.

Fran, C., Dasaklisb Thomas, K., Constantinos, P. 2018. A systematic literature review of blockchain-based applications: Current status, classification and open issues. *Telematics and Informatics*, Published by Elsevier Ltd. Available online: journal homepage: www. elsevier.com/locate/tele.

Gendal. 2015. Available online: http://gendal.me/2015/07/23/bitcoin-and-blockchain-two-revolutions-for-the-price-of-one (accessed on 31 December 2021).

Ho, P.J., Hyuk, P.J. 2017. Blockchain security in cloud computing: Use cases, challenges, and solutions. *Symmetry*, 9, 164. Available online: www.mdpi.com/journal/symmetry.

Idrees, S.M., Nowostawski, M., Jameel, R. 2021a. Blockchain-based digital contact tracing apps for COVID-19 pandemic management: Issues, challenges, solutions, and future directions. *JMIR Medical Informatics*, 9(2), e25245.

Idrees, S.M., Nowostawski, M., Jameel, R., Mourya, A.K. 2021. Security Aspects of Blockchain Technology Intended for Industrial Applications. Electronics 2021, 10, 951. https://doi.org/10.3390/electronics10080951

Idrees, S.M., Nowostawski, M., Jameel, R., Mourya, A.K. 2021b. 7 privacy-preserving. In *Data Protection and Privacy in Healthcare: Research and Innovations*, CRC Press: Boca Raton, FL, p. 109.

Julija, G., Andrejs, R. 2018. The advantages and disadvantages of the blockchain technology, IEEE.

Jun, L., Alex, G., Jeremy, K., Charles, F. 2020. LBRY: A blockchain-based decentralized digital content marketplace. *IEEE International Conference on Decentralized Applications and Infrastructures (DAPPS)*, IEEE Xplore Oxford, U.K.

Liu, C., Xu, X., Hu, D.2015. Multiobjective reinforcement learning: A comprehensive overview. *IEEE Transactions on Systems, Man, and Cybernetics: Systems*, 45(3), 385–398.

MongoDB. Accessed: January 4, 2021. [Online]. Available: https://www.mongodb.com/.

Morgen, P., et al., 2017. Reinforcing the links of the blockchain. *IEEE Future Directions Blockchain Initiative White Paper Blockchain Incubator*, Available online: www.IEEE.ORG.

Qiu, C., Yu, F.R., Xu, F., Yao, H., Zhao, C. 2018. Blockchain-based distributed software-defined vehicular networks via deep Q-learning, *In Proceedings of 8th ACM Symposium Design and Analysis of Intelligent Vehicular Networks and Applications*, New York, pp. 8–14.

Redis. (2019). Accessed: December 28, 2020. [Online]. Available: https://redis.io/.

Salah, K., Rehman, M.H.U., Nizamuddin, N., Al-Fuqaha, A. 2019. Blockchain for ai: Review and open research challenges. *IEEE Access*, 7, 10127–10149.

Seyednima, K., Md, M., Abdulsalam, Y., Benlamri, R. 2019. Blockchain technology in healthcare: A comprehensive review and directions for future research. Licensee MDPI, Basel, Switzerland. *Applied Sciences*, 9, 1736. doi:10.3390/app9091736, Available online: www.mdpi.com/journal/applsci.

Srinivas, K., Reddy, M.P.K., Gautam, S. 2020. Deep learning disease prediction model for use with intelligent robots. *Computers and Electrical Engineering*, 87, 106765.

Tanesh, K., Vidhya, R., Ijaz, A., An, B., Erkki, H., Mika, Y. 2018.Blockchain utilization in healthcare: Key requirements and challenges. *IEEE 20th International Conference on e-Health Networking, Applications and Services (Healthcom) Ostrava, CzechRepublic*.

Vapnik, V. 1995. *The Nature of Statistical Learning Theory*. Springer: Berlin/Heidelberg.

Velankar, S., Valecha, S., Maji, S. 2018. Bitcoin price prediction using machine learning, *20th International Conference on Advanced Communication Technology (ICACT)*, South Korea, pp. 144–147.

Wang, W.M., Guo, H., Li, Z., Shen, Y., Barenji, A.V. 2018. Towards automated customer service: A blockchain based auto ML framework. *2018 Association for Computing Machinery*. ACM, ISBN 978-1-4503-6512, March 18, 2018.

Wasim, M.U., Ibrahim, A.A.Z.A., Bouvry, P., Limba, T. 2017. Law as a service (LAAS): Enabling legal protection over a blockchain network, *In 2017 14th International Conference on Smart Cities: Improving Quality of Life Using ICT & IoT (HONET-ICT)*, Irvid/ Amman, Jordan, October 2017, pp. 110–114.

Zhou, Y., et al., 2018. Huawei blockchain whitepaper.

9 Blockchain-based Solutions for COVID-19

Challenges, Advantages, and Applications

Neha and Pooja Gupta
Jamia Hamdard

CONTENTS

DOI: 10.1201/9781003141471-9

9.1   INTRODUCTION OF BLOCKCHAIN IN HEALTHCARE

The coronavirus (COVID-19) outbreak, an acute respiratory disease caused by the SARS-CoV2, gave rise to a worldwide health emergency in 2020. The family of coronaviruses can cause illnesses like the common flu, severe acute respiratory syndrome (SARS), and the Middle East respiratory syndrome (MERS), and they are transmitted through respiratory droplets, making them extremely fatal. The WHO declared the COVID-19 outbreak as a pandemic, owing to the extent of deaths it caused across the world.

While the virus affected the health of people, it had an equal impact on their lives in general and more so on the global economy. A number of countries resorted to restrictive measures like complete lockdowns in order to try to keep a check on the pandemic. As a result, half of the total population of the world was restricted to leave their homes by early April followed by a temporary closure of most factories, markets, and businesses which ultimately engendered an extreme economic slowdown.

Although governments and researchers across the world have been working vivaciously to find a cure, the sudden outburst of the pandemic has exposed the shortcomings in contemporary healthcare systems. Utilizing ingenious technologies like blockchain can prove out to be really advantageous in a situation this vulnerable. Blockchain technology can really be functional in revamping the healthcare systems by facilitating a smooth clinical trial data management, foreshortening the processing time, and rationalizing a fair communication between multiple stakeholders of the supply chain.

A blockchain is based on the concept of peer-to-peer connectivity with a distributed consensus-based mechanism. Decentralization, transparency, and autonomy are some of its features [1] (Figure 9.1).

Blockchain is basically a chain of logically connected blocks [4]. Each block contains the information of the previous block in hashed format and a time-stamp. A transaction has to be performed in the network in order to create a new block. All the participants in the network get to know about this transaction which has to be verified by participants also called miners. After the verification is done successfully, a new block is created and is linked to the blockchain [1].

The distributed consensus-based framework of blockchain ensures secure exchange of information without the supervision of any central authority. This can

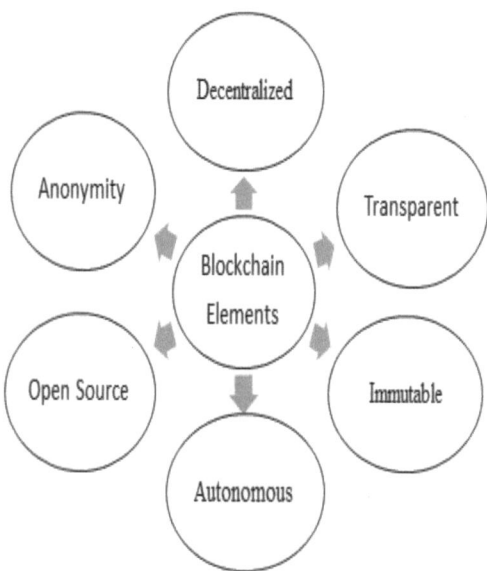

FIGURE 9.1 Key elements of blockchain.

be utilized in the healthcare sector for managing and processing data and hence is apt to handle the healthcare situations arising due to COVID-19. In addition, blockchain can be utilized to curb the fake news that has increased during this outbreak. This will guarantee that the information reaching people is genuine.

Blockchain can be integrated into the healthcare system for its fight against COVID-19 as it facilitates tracking and managing supply chain and security of data. It can play a pivotal role in delivering a solution that is transparent and reliable as well as can quickly intervene to deter this crisis.

9.2 GENERAL CHALLENGES FACED DURING COVID-19 PANDEMIC

The COVID-19 flare-up in late 2019 caused a worldwide medical crisis. In a little more than a quarter of a year, the quantity of COVID new cases has risen to in excess of 1,000,000 around the world. The fast transmission of the infection prompts new cases to be accounted for all around the world constantly. At the same time, mortality rate and contaminations keep on rising rapidly. Therefore, the COVID-19 pandemic has led to the implementation of lockdowns and social distancing rules that negatively impact global economies. It has upturned many challenges which are mentioned in this section [5,6] (Figure 9.2).

9.2.1 DISINFODEMIC

Due to the improper description of this spreading virus and the lack of drugs, a domain has been developed with huge spurious information. It activates self-medication, which sometimes develops other health problems. It also causes psychosomatic disorders. It

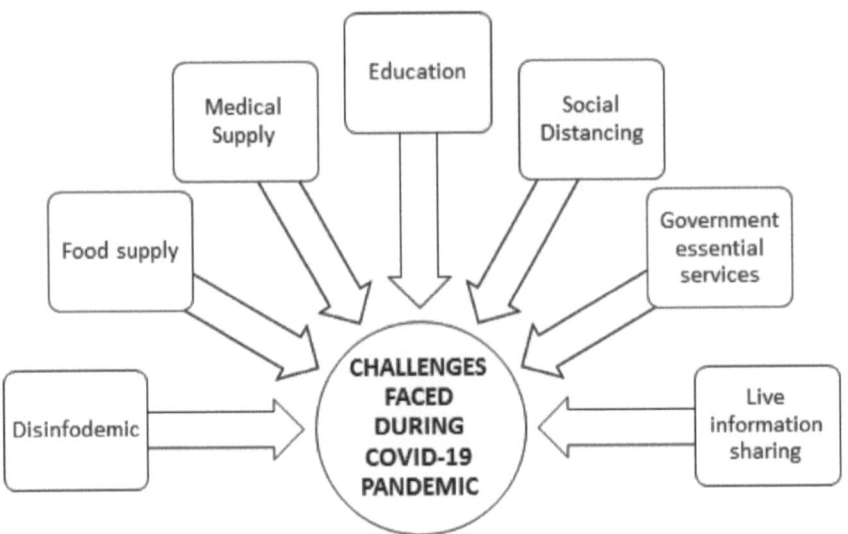

FIGURE 9.2 Significant challenges during COVID-19.

has also been observed that a sudden stop in normal life (i.e., restrictions in movements, working, and socialization) increases anxiety and stress.

Furthermore, the development of a predicted model and estimation on future demands based on such information would be incoherent concurrent platforms, and their underlying technologies cannot deal with this problem and counterfeit information is becoming harder to counter.

9.2.2 FOOD SUPPLY

Due to the outbreak of coronavirus, many nations have called for a complete lockdown. Limited transport services also affect the food supply chain. It creates a misbalance state in demand and supply as the situation influences both consumers and producers. Many people are encountering starvation as they have lost their means of livelihood. Concurrently, agronomists of agriculture-dependent nations are suffering in order to sell their products. In this manner, there is a standstill state in the agrarian area.

9.2.3 MEDICAL SUPPLY

This rampant virus caused medical pressure all over the world. There is a massive requirement of medical supplies globally like masks, sanitizers, face shields, ventilators, personal protective equipment (PPE) kits, testing kits, and so on. Timely delivery of these supplies is quite tedious without a suitable supply chain and inventory. India additionally offers more than 20% of generic drugs to different nations [7]. As there is no existing medical structure to combat this disease, some sellers may block the accessibility of essential medical products to artificially inflate prices. Besides, there is a high probability of quality compromises and counterfeit products.

9.2.4 EDUCATION

Educational sectors also witness the coronavirus. Educational institutions of several nations are also closed during this lockdown period. However, the education sector has switched to digital technologies in this phase. The instantaneous adaptation of online education modes shoots up the data traffic in the existing internet infrastructures. Despite the fact that online platforms have been embraced, it includes some technical issues like lack of proper web infrastructures, heavy data flow, and unavailability of trained educators. The effective teaching-learning technique has been hampered due to lack of some vital dimensions like real-time discussions, gesture, and concentration in students. Other security flaws have also been accounted for some online platforms like Zoom conferencing [6,9].

9.2.5 SOCIAL DISTANCING

Since there is no drugs or vaccine available, the practice of social distancing is imposed to break the chain of viruses and "flatten the curve" of fresh cases. Also, several physical interactions are suspended during the lockdown. Restricted interactions results in social isolation and adverse psychological effects.

9.2.6 GOVERNMENT ESSENTIAL SERVICES

Several services like tax collection, pension, salary, birth/death registration, and public utilities are relied upon to be accessible consistently. However continuous operation and delivery of these services become tough as public authorities are also bound by the lockdown norms.

9.2.7 LIVE INFORMATION SHARING

Worldwide information synchronization is a basic factor in fighting the COVID-19 pandemic. In India, the government has launched the Arogya Setu mobile app, which provides an assessment of the number of infected people, active cases, recovery of patients, etc. It also keeps a record of the movement of individuals and alerts them by knowing nearby real-time data. Sharing important information makes immediate proactive action helpful to create public awareness and predict future patterns though digital data sharing tends to security and privacy attacks. In the absence of proper security standards, data may tamper and mishandle.

9.3 BLOCKCHAIN IN HEALTHCARE SECTOR: PROMISING USE CASES FOR BLOCKCHAIN TECHNOLOGY IN HEALTHCARE

The conventional technologies used in the healthcare ecosystem pose many challenges like privacy, security, interoperability, and data tampering. Blockchain with its secure distributed ledger technique can handle several such challenges. Following are a few areas in healthcare industry where blockchain technology can prove beneficial [10].

9.3.1 Drug Traceability

One of the major issues in the healthcare industry is that of counterfeit drugs. These drugs contain different ingredients than that of the original drug. Also, there are cases where correct ingredients are used but they are in the wrong proportion. Hence, they may not perform their intended task and can have side effects as well.

Blockchain can help in solving this crucial problem by providing the facility of tracking right from the production of drugs till they reach the end-user. This will curb their presence in the market and will allow the stakeholders to keep a watch over the entire supply chain.

9.3.2 Clinical Trials

Clinical trials are performed to test the efficacy of a drug, which involves a considerable amount of time. In addition to the long-drawn process, an enormous number of people are involved in clinical trials. This produces a large amount of data handling which with the help of conventional techniques involves various issues like privacy, security, and data theft. Blockchain can be used effectively to handle all such issues.

9.3.3 Patient Data Management

Patient data management is a highly sensitive part of the healthcare system, and the exchange of this information is regulated. Access to complete medical history is required to provide the correct course of treatment. Blockchain technology can be used here to facilitate the secure exchange of data. It can also be used to allow patients to have control over their medical records and the accessing entity.

9.4 BLOCKCHAIN AND COVID-19: HOW COVID-19 HAS REVEALED HEALTHCARE'S BLOCKCHAIN USE CASES

Blockchain technology is known for its qualities of decentralization, privacy, and transparency. In the wake of COVID-19 pandemic, several functionalities in the healthcare sector have emerged where blockchain technology can prove beneficial. Following are few such use cases [2,3,20].

9.4.1 Contact Tracing

To curb the spread of the novel coronavirus, governments throughout the world have undertaken the strategy of contact tracing. In this, an infected person lists out everybody who has come in his/her contact so that they can be isolated, hence checking further transmissions. Blockchain along with other technologies such as artificial intelligence and global positioning system can track the movement of infected people without disclosing their identity. It can provide case information of the surrounding areas. Also, since the data collected is very sensitive and involves privacy concerns, blockchain with its features of accuracy and reliability can be used here effectively (Figure 9.3).

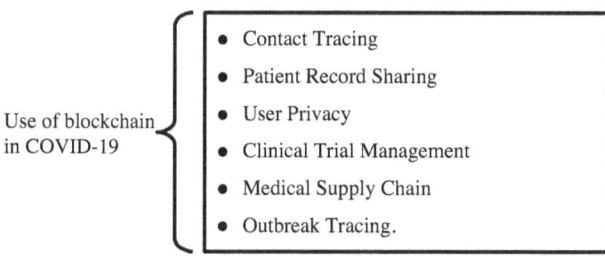

Use of blockchain in COVID-19
- Contact Tracing
- Patient Record Sharing
- User Privacy
- Clinical Trial Management
- Medical Supply Chain
- Outbreak Tracing.

FIGURE 9.3   Use of blockchain in COVID-19.

9.4.2 PATIENT RECORD SHARING

The idea here is to store the health records of patients in electronic format and to share them digitally [2]. During the pandemic, these health records can be aggregated and shared. This will allow healthcare providers to access the medical history of a patient with whom they are not familiar at all and the patients to get medical help no matter where they are. Blockchain can be used for these functionalities while ensuring the accuracy and integrity of data. It can be used to monitor the symptoms and follow the advancements of a patient.

The aggregation of information is also required to find out the infection trail, interpret trends, and spearhead the research in the right direction. The distributed ledger framework of blockchain can aid in the exchange of research data among stakeholders so that research and development of new solutions go on at the same pace while taking feedback from each other [3].

9.4.3 USER PRIVACY

Ever since the pandemic started, governments have been collecting data about the patients for various purposes necessary for curbing the infection. Protecting this data is very important to avoid any privacy breach.

Blockchain can solve this purpose of data collection on one hand and identity protection of patients on the other as it allows a person to have control over their data. So, they can choose to share only that part of information that is relevant to the COVID-19 [11].

9.4.4 CLINICAL TRIAL MANAGEMENT

An efficient and transparent management system is essentially required for clinical trials to operate systematically. The application of digital technologies in this field can be very helpful in order to provide safety and privacy to the participants, while at the same time narrowing down the trial timelines up to a great extent [6]. Blockchain technology can provide a valuable assistance to researchers and practitioners in real-time documentation of clinical data, thereby improving data precision, facilitating information exchange, and fulfilling statutory requirements. It can also track and maintain a record of the accessed part of the datasets, thus aiding to improve data protection.

9.4.5 MEDICAL SUPPLY CHAIN

The COVID-19 epidemic has interrupted the supply chains across the whole world tremendously, because of the shutting down of numerous factories, and an unprecedented increase in the demand for certain products like the PPE [6,8].

Blockchain has emerged as the most suited option for supply chains, for one simple fact that it can adhere all collaborators into a single supply chain network while at the same time strengthening transparency and securely dismantling data silos. An added advantage is the reduction in processing time, costs, and operational risks substantially for all stakeholders.

9.4.6 OUTBREAK TRACING

Unverified data creates a lot of chaos and causes economic and psychological damage. A blockchain database puts a check on the modification of data and makes any alteration detectable, thereby facilitating an easy way to avoid fake information.

Thus, blockchain technology has proved to be a spreading coronavirus tracking platform as data is handled through it, reliable, and transparent. Governments and authorities can use it to update more efficiently on the status of the coronavirus pandemic, paving a way for an advanced scheming of things and better management.

9.5 ADVANTAGES OF BLOCKCHAIN TECHNOLOGY FOR COVID-19

Blockchain maintains security and privacy of the information. A section in this chapter also covers the feasible ways of this technology in combating COVID-19 situations. In addition to transparency, accuracy, and consistency in storage of information, blockchain holds the following comprehensive properties [4,12]:

1. **Architectural Aspects**: Architectural features means peer-to-peer transmission, encrypted data, secured data distribution, and transmission.
2. **Logical Inclusion**: It mentions transaction protocol, computational logic, and transactional dependency.
3. **Service Approach**: This ensures scalability, validity, and reliability of the data.

It can therefore bring an improvement for the section where centralization is simulated and security and privacy are important. It can be used everywhere to follow the spread of the virus. An important advantage of this technique is the preservation of patient data. It also simplifies complicated medical setup process and eliminates third parties. Patients can upload and secure their medical records safely. These digital records of patients can be accessible by authorized bodies only. This can keep a record for upcoming vaccines and drug trials as well as mobility control, monitor the medical funds and grants, and bring transparency to the developing system.

9.6 PROBLEMS IN THE ADAPTATION OF BLOCKCHAIN IN HEALTHCARE

Though this technology has many pros still, it encounters enormous challenges. A couple of these significant difficulties are mentioned in this segment. Figure 9.4 depicts some concerning areas in the adaptation of blockchain technology [1,13,14].

9.6.1 SUSTAINABILITY

All information is encrypted in this technology. Hence encryption keys have significance in the blockchain. There is no way to retrieve private encrypted keys. This brings complexity to health data due to its enduring nature. If a patient's data is missed or lost , its reliability and value inevitably decreases. In addition, if the user's private encryption key is snooped, it allows access to all stored information.

9.6.2 TRANSPARENCY AND PRIVACY

Security is another important subject here. Transparency might not be mandatory in every case for the health care domain. Despite the fact that it gives security through encryption, accessibility of information is a significant challenge for medical service partners. Subsequently, access control with regard to blockchain must be handled appropriately.

9.6.3 SCALABILITY

The significant technology concern is its technical scalability of the network, which can fade the adaption process. With the addition of new data, blockchain network needs expansion in storage and computational power. If medical professionals fail to meet any of these demands, the ability to centralize and slow data validation and validation increases.

9.6.4 LIMITED STORAGE CAPACITY

Another adaptability issue is about a decent storage capacity. The purpose of the blockchain was intended to record and handle the transaction, which has a restricted range, so it doesn't need much capacity [15]. Over time when the blockchain network

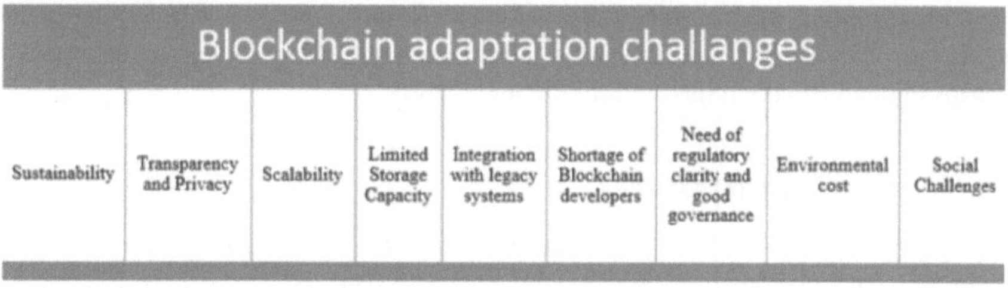

Blockchain adaptation challanges								
Sustainability	Transparency and Privacy	Scalability	Limited Storage Capacity	Integration with legacy systems	Shortage of Blockchain developers	Need of regulatory clarity and good governance	Environmental cost	Social Challenges

FIGURE 9.4 Challenges in blockchain adaptation.

expands in health services, area storage will also become a barrier. In the medical field, tremendous data has to be processed consistently. From patients' medical history, pathological reports to all medical images (e.g., MRI, X-rays, CT scan, and ultrasound) will be accessible to all hubs in the chain, which demand a huge repository. Database is widened day by day. Hence the access rate seems to be slowing down, which is also undesirable and unsatisfactory.

9.6.5 Integration with Legacy Systems

The challenge before the healthcare system is how to coordinate blockchain with the traditional medical infrastructure system. If they choose to adopt blockchain, the existing infrastructure has to be completely restructured or plan another approach for effective coordination. As few skilled blockchain developers are available, many organizations need to perform in collaboration, although this accelerates the adoption of blockchain and simultaneously expands the dependency and risk of data breaches. Interfacing existing medical services with blockchain backend may help in this problem. Another approach to solve this issue is the Modex blockchain database. It is a product intended to help people without prior knowledge of technology and to access the advantages of blockchain. Additionally, it eliminates threats presented by the breach of sensitive information.

9.6.6 Shortage of Blockchain Developers

Blockchain innovation is still in an emerging state. It needs time for the developer community to embrace it. Due to this pandemic, there is an urgent call for upgradation in the healthcare sector. The demand for qualified developers is expanding significantly, the blockchain scene endures an intense shortfall of trained employees to manage and deal with the complexity of the network.

9.6.7 Need Regulatory Clarity and Good Governance

There is also insufficient interoperability among the blockchain networks. The proposed blockchain-based health care system requires interfacing in public and private blockchain. It increases the need for proper coordination, standards, and regulations globally. There is a shortage of such regulatory bodies and standards, which is a critical route for mass-level adoption. Some areas like smart contracts must need proper regulations. Government and higher authorities may have to make guidelines for blockchain. However, this implies that controllers in the medical services area need to comprehend the technology and its effect [1,14].

9.6.8 Environmental Cost

Massive energy consumption is another blockchain adoption challenge. Most blockchains exist, which consume high amounts of energy. Bitcoin infrastructure is followed to approve transactions. These protocols require users to solve complex mathematical puzzles and require tremendous computing power to certify transactions and secure

Strength	Weakness	Opportunities	Threats
• Tamper-Evident data sharing. • Quick access to medical data. • Cost effective	• Shortages of trained Blockchain developers • Unavailability of software and system assistance. • Insufficient Storage Capacity	• Confidentiality of data boost Medical researches. • Minimize fraud risk in the medical supply chain. • Wide opening for start-ups,patnerships and collabratios.	• Cultural and trust concern to accept Blockchain for sensitive data. • Interoperabiity concerns • Non standardization • Reluctant social adoption.

FIGURE 9.5   Analysis for blockchain in healthcare.

networks [15]. To overcome this problem, many blockchain developers are developing more efficient algorithms, which are energy efficient.

9.6.9 Social Challenges

Blockchain also faces some social challenges. It may be due to the lack of awareness and proper understanding of the technology. Welcoming and embracing a new technology is not so easy for society. In spite of the fact that healthcare domain is gradually shifted toward digitization, there is still a gap in full adoption of blockchain. Persuading medical specialists to change from conventional paperwork to adopt this technology will require some serious energy and effort. For better understanding, the strength, weakness, opportunities, and threat analysis [15] for blockchain in healthcare are illustrated in Figure 9.5.

9.7 APPLICATION OF BLOCKCHAIN TECHNOLOGY IN COMBATING COVID-19

Before discussing the potential methods to implement blockchain to deal with this virus, we enlisted few domains facing problems due to this contagious virus as:

1. How the existing health care systems are prepared to counter this outburst.
2. Monitor and control infectious patients to prevent the epidemic.
3. Deception and paranoid fears outspread through several platforms like social media.
4. There is an urgent need to develop a better diagnosis, vaccines, and targeted therapeutics.
5. No satisfactory measures to embrace in an emergency circumstance.
6. Several restrictions.

The blockchain is tamper-proof ledger technology. Blockchain can set up a reliable, transparent, and accurate healthcare framework. This technology helps us to develop an edge of protection. The primary goal of blockchain-enabled networks is to be

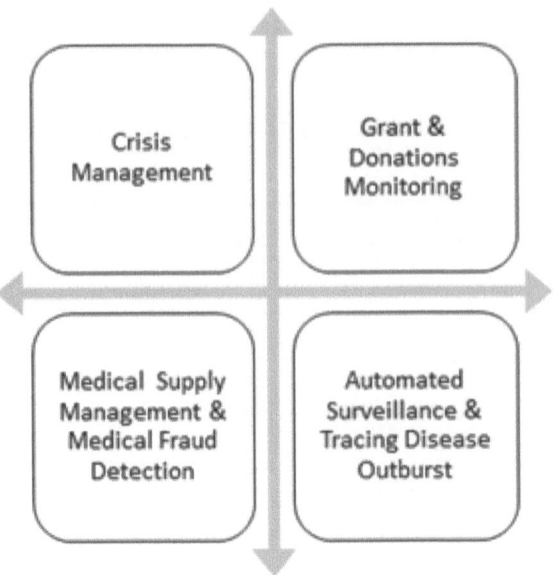

FIGURE 9.6 Blockchain applications in combating COVID-19.

vigilant about disease outbreaks [16]. Consequently, the blockchain adopted health models could be more informative about drug trials, early diagnosis of virus, testing, and impact management of outburst and treatment. For this situation, there was a blockchain where WHO, Ministry of Health, and relevant hospitals of all nations associated sharing real-time data on the contagious disease. Blockchain application in combating COVID-19 is shown in Figure 9.6.

9.7.1 CRISIS MANAGEMENT

In 1994, Nick Szabo first termed the "Smart contract" concept. It is a tamper-proof, self-executed, self-verified computer program. The basic structure of smart contract is shown in Figure 9.7. Basically, a smart contract consists of the value, address, functions, and state. It accepts transaction as an information, executes the comparing code, and stimulates output [17].

The significance of smart contract integration with blockchain offers peer-to-peer transactions. Additionally, the database can be conserved in a reliable and safe

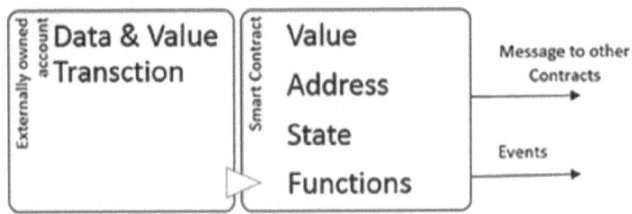

FIGURE 9.7 Basic Structure of Smart Contract

manner. Smart contracts are trackable and immutable. Smart contracts are distributed, and machine legible codes run on blockchain platforms. Blockchain-based smart contracts can provide various advantages [18,19]:

1. Precision
2. Live and fast updates.
3. Minimize third-party interference.
4. Reduction in execution threats.
5. Scope of new business models.
6. Budget-friendly setups.

Blockchain provides a secure forum where all scrutinizing authorities can notify everyone regarding the condition and suppress it from deteriorating further. It can be used as a virus vigilance tool.

9.7.2 GRANT AND DONATIONS MONITORING

Reliability is a concerning factor in grants and donations. A major concern is to ensure appropriate distribution and maintain transparency to the contributors. Hence a system is required to develop trust and for proper monitoring of funds and donations. Blockchain has ability to meet this requirement. Blockchain integrated system aids transparency and helps in the monitoring of funds. Blockchain provides the ease to trace the complete process: from the release of funds or collection of donations to its utilization and progress. The contributors can see where the money is needed, and they can follow their contributions until they are verified that the victims have received their contribution.

9.7.3 MEDICAL SUPPLY MANAGEMENT AND FRAUD DETECTION

Because of this virus, many nations call off all types of movements. It interrupts the various ongoing supply chains. Demands of the products are based on their type. For example due to panic buying, the demand for essential items (food, medicine, etc.) increased. Likewise, clinical hardware and drug supply chains are also facing difficulties to fulfill the serious need. In this case, blockchain technology can be significant in developing and managing the more flexible supply chain. The blockchain-based system can be convenient in evaluating, tracking, and tracing the demand and supplies. As many parties are involved in supply chains, the complete cycle of documentation and verification is sealed by every party. Furthermore, anyone can follow the cycle. Blockchain-driven cross-country data sharing approaches can deal with immigration and emigration processes efficiently. Moreover, this streamlined medical chain also confirms the reach of medical apparatus to doctors and patients as per their requirements and forbids contaminated things from reaching stores.

Apart from medical supplies management, it can be implemented to observe medical frauds. Supply chain involves various people and operational sections that make it prone to attacks and frauds. Blockchain establishes a secure platform for operation. It upscales data transparency and boosts product tracking in the system.

It is not easy to manipulate the blockchain, since the information in the blockchain is validated and streamlined via a smart contract only.

9.7.4 AUTOMATED SURVEILLANCE AND TRACING DISEASE OUTBREAKS

Face masks, frequently washing hands, sanitization, social distancing, contactless deliveries, self-health assessment (by using authorized official apps), etc. are adopted as precautionary measures in COVID-19 situations. Nonetheless, embracing these practices looks to be burdensome as people are not used to them. It raises the need for steady and automated surveillance for cautions. For such conditions, blockchain-enabled unmanned aerial vehicles (UAVs) are adopted. UAVs carry out functions without human involvement. Hence, it can be employed for several exercises like surveillance, contactless delivery, and testing. Blockchain accompanying smart contracts can engage UAVs for reliable operation. It gives confined access to record information and incorporates contactless payment or digital payment methods.

Blockchain enhances transparency, and this will bring highly precise and systematic reporting and responses. It can accelerate the drug invention process as they would consider fast data processing, accordingly empowering early diagnosis of symptoms before they spread to the degree of pandemics. Also, this will empower authorized offices to monitor the virus graph, patient movement, and suspected new cases [6,16,18].

9.8 CONCLUSION

COVID-19 has wreaked havoc all over the world. Almost all sectors are negatively affected, such as healthcare, education, and the economy. There are various challenges that arise while using the conventional techniques for tackling such pandemics. Blockchain can be used to overcome these issues. In this chapter, we have explored the areas in the healthcare sector where blockchain can be of use. The vulnerability caused by the COVID-19 pandemic has indicated the need to develop a single blockchain-based healthcare and management system to address many current and future problems. We have explained several such use cases such as contact tracing, patient record sharing, user privacy, clinical trial management, etc. that can be implemented successfully using the basic features of blockchain. Despite all these plus points, there are some concerns and challenges associated with this technology. We have mentioned a few such problematic areas in this chapter. In addition, we have discussed the advantages and application areas of blockchain in COVID-19.

REFERENCES

1. Siyal, A. A., Junejo, A. Z., Zawish, M., Ahmed, K., Khalil, A., & Soursou, G. (2019). Applications of blockchain technology in medicine and healthcare: Challenges and future perspectives. *Cryptography, 3*(1), 3.
2. https://hitconsultant.net/2020/11/17/covid-19-healthcare-blockchain-use-cases/#.X-NlG1UzbIX.
3. Marbouh, D., Abbasi, T., Maasmi, F., Omar, I. A., Debe, M. S., Salah, K., ... & Ellahham, S. (2020). Blockchain for COVID-19: Review, opportunities, and a trusted tracking system. *Arabian Journal for Science and Engineering, 45*(12), 1–17.

4. Islam, I., Munim, K. M., Oishwee, S. J., Islam, A. N., & Islam, M. N. (2020). A critical review of concepts, benefits, and pitfalls of blockchain technology using concept map. *IEEE Access, 8*, 68333–68341.

5. World Health Organization (WHO). Rolling updates on coronavirus disease (COVID-19). https://www.who.int/emergencies/diseases/novel-coronavirus-2019/events-as-they-happen.

6. Kalla, A., Hewa, T., Mishra, R. A., Ylianttila, M., & Liyanage, M. (2020). The role of blockchain to fight against COVID-19. *IEEE Engineering Management Review, 48*(3), 85–96.

7. Annual Report 2019–20, Ministry of Chemicals and Fertilizers, Department of Pharmaceuticals, accessed on 06.06.2020. Online. Available: https://pharmaceuticals.gov.in/sites/default/files/Annual\%20Report\%202019-20.pdf.

8. Guerin, P. J., Singh-Phulgenda, S., & Strub-Wourgaft, N. (2020). The consequence of COVID-19 on the global supply of medical products: Why Indian generics matter for the world? F1000Research, 9(225), 225.

9. Aiken, A. (2020). Zooming in on privacy concerns, *Index on Censorship*, 49(2), 24–27. doi: 10.1177/0306422020935792.

10. https://innovationatwork.ieee.org/3-promising-use-cases-for-blockchain-technology-in-healthcare/.

11. Dragov, R., Croce, C. L., & Hefny, M. (2020). How blockchain can help in the COVID-19 crisis and recovery. IDC-Analyze the Future, May 4.

12. Azim, A., Islam, M. N., & Spranger, P. E. (2020). Blockchain and novel coronavirus: Towards preventing COVID-19 and future pandemics. *Iberoamerican Journal of Medicine*, 2(3), 215–218. (Ahead of Print).

13. Gökalp, E., Gökalp, M. O., Çoban, S., & Eren, P. E. (2018, September). Analysing opportunities and challenges of integrated blockchain technologies in healthcare. In *EuroSymposium on Systems Analysis and Design* (pp. 174–183). Springer, Cham.

14. https://www.finextra.com/blogposting/18496/remaining-challenges-of-blockchain-adoption-and-possible-solutions.

15. Esposito, C., De Santis, A., Tortora, G., Chang, H., & Choo, K. K. R. (2018). Blockchain: A panacea for healthcare cloud-based data security and privacy? *IEEE Cloud Computing*, 5(1), 31–37.

16. https://www.bbvaopenmind.com/en/technology/digital-world/blockchain-technology-and-covid-19/.

17. Szabo, N. (1997). Formalizing and securing relationships on public networks. *First Monday*, 2(9). doi: 10.5210/fm.v2i9.548.

18. https://www.blockchain-council.org/blockchain/how-blockchain-can-solve-major-challenges-of-covid-19-faced-by-healthcare-sectors/.

19. Mohanta, B., Panda, S., & Jena, D. (2018). An overview of smart contract and use cases in blockchain technology. 2018 9th International Conference on Computing, Communication and Networking Technologies (ICCCNT), 1–4. IEEE, Bengaluru.

20. Idrees, S. M., Nowostawski, M., & Jameel, R. (2021). Blockchain-based digital contact tracing apps for COVID-19 pandemic management: Issues, challenges, solutions, and future directions. *JMIR Medical Informatics*, 9(2), e25245.

10 Managing Medical Supply Chain Using Blockchain Technology

Ihtiram Raza Khan and Mohd Adnan Baig
Jamia Hamdard

CONTENTS

10.1 INTRODUCTION

Flow of different goods, flow of information, and flow of services between different entities of that particular business cycle demand a secure network. In every industry, poor supply chain is an open invitation for many major issues but there is an additional risk of patient's health in healthcare sector. Healthcare industry requires optimized solutions that can smooth different operations and processes of supply chain [1]. As in healthcare sector compromise with a fragile supply chain is nothing but compromise with the patient's health, the extent to which a pharmaceutical organization disregards the security in the business supply chain is directly proportional to the intensity of health risk. Among various other challenges in pharmaceutical business, delivering an original product (medicine) to the consumer after a long process of drug formulation, clinical trials, and final development is a big one. If we look in the light of recent COVID-19 pandemic, the presence of more manpower holds a risk of fast spread of virus [2].

DOI: 10.1201/9781003141471-10

In present system of supply chain in pharma industry every component whether they are manufacturer, distributor, or any other component, everyone is working on their own methods and systems for management of flow and manufacturing of medicines [3].

Lack of visibility in a supply chain raises many questions like how a manufacturing firm will know about the raw materials requirement, and tracing of goods stored in warehouse in semi-finished and finished form as in a multi-layered supply chain management of inventory is an important factor to be taken in account. If a manufacturer and a distributor don't have a clear vision about raw materials present, raw materials required, and quantity of semi-finished and finished goods, all these factors lead to inefficient inventory management which results in many problems such as the problem of understocking, overstocking, wastage of resources, less profit, cost increment, and imbalancement of overall business flow. If we talk about pharma industry, India has emerged as a leading, dominant, and wide pharmaceutical industry in terms of volume in the world [4]. India's exportation of drugs has increased from 6.23 US billion dollars in 2006–2007 to 8.7 US billion dollars in 2008–2009[5]. However, all these loop holes discussed are major causes of drug shortages [6]. So in order to avoid the issue of drug shortage, drug managers should have a clear vision about the availability of inventory for the production of medicines at their end. How a distributor will know about the source of asked drugs whether they are coming from authorized source or from some other malicious intermediate entity. Among 10 drugs, 1 drug is fake or substandard [7]. According to a WHO report 20 million pills, bottles of falsified medicines were seized in Egypt during a raid in 2009 in Egypt by ICPO [8]. These counterfeited drugs contain toxic ingredients and many times active ingredients either in incorrect measure or in impure manner, which deals with the health of patients abruptly. After intake, even original medicine fails to work properly in some cases [9]. Counterfeiting also violates intellectual property rights. How two entities will get to know about the location of a patched medicine during transportation? How a consumer will know the details about medicine, like its actual price, date of manufacturing, date of expiry, and so on to be ensured about the authenticity of medicine. All these security features are missing from the existing system of supply chain in the healthcare sector.

Cold chain shipping of drugs, which are temperature sensitive, can lose their potential when exposed to hot temperature is an additional issue. Cold chain refers to the normal distribution of goods in a standard supply chain but with controlled humidity and temperature [10]. Out of 50 drugs, 26 need to be shipped through cold chain [11]. All these problems like proper inventory management in order to scale up with market's demand –shifting data gathered by IoT sensors during cold chain shipping, and last but not least, that is counterfeiting –can be solved by the transparent nature of blockchain technology. Blockchain among existing ledger systems on the planet is considered as one of the most secured ones [9]. Blockchain is defined as the network of connected systems called blocks. Each block of blockchain technology represents a set of information. Every entity in a blockchain network will have a copy of each block. And all of them will be aware of all transactions going on. So whenever a new block is added or updated, it will require verification from other entities in the network, and only after verification process, person can access the information. So use of this technology for managing supply chain will provide a network where every component will be aware of all transactions, like information about the manufacturer, drugs sources and its movement in between, and blockchain for traceability along with IoT for cold chain shipping. This way blockchain puts efforts in maintaining visibility and traceability.

10.2 PROBLEM STATEMENT

There are numerous problems in the existing system of supply chain in the healthcare sector; some of them are listed below [11].

10.2.1 COUNTERFEITING OF DRUGS

Counterfeiting of drugs is emerging as the biggest challenge for the pharma industry to tackle around the globe. Counterfeiting refers to the illegal process of formation of duplicate goods in the name of legitimate good. They enter in the pre-established business supply chain through the loopholes present in it. A counterfeit drug is a medicine which either doesn't contain proper dosage or contain in an improper manner. Counterfeiting of medicines is a criminal offence as it atrociously deals with patient's health. According to WHO among 1 million deaths from malaria per year, 0.2% of them was the result of falsified drugs [9]. In developing countries, 30% of the total drugs sold are fake [9].The sale of fake drugs has been increased from 75 billion US dollars in 2009 to 600 billion US dollars in 2018 [8]. These falsified drugs enter the supply chain mostly during transportation between different entities due to the lack of traceability in the present system.

10.2.2 COUNTERFEITING (THREAT TO IPR)

Counterfeiters use logos of legitimate manufacturers in many cases, which violate intellectual property rights and IP laws. Also making a fake drug means using someone's innovation without their consent which is illegal.

10.2.3 LOSS OF LEGITIMATE MANUFACTURERS

Counterfeiting of drugs is not harmful only for consumers but also for legitimate manufacturers. Production of original medicine requires more resources and manpower and involves cost as compared to the production of falsified drugs. In addition, it is easier to sell fake drugs. In US pharmaceutical industry, fake drugs caused a total loss of 200 billion US dollars [7].

10.2.4 DRUG SHORTAGE

Drug shortage problem arises due to the lack of visibility in the pharma supply chain in the present system. Many times, it is quite difficult for inventory managers to keep track of market demand, cost of manufacturing, time required to produce a final medicine, quantity of raw material, and different types of goods developed. When these factors result in understocking, this leads to drug shortage in the market.

10.2.5 SENSITIVE DRUG SHIPPING

Sensitive shipping is also known as cold chain shipping. Cold chain shipping is defined as the shipping of goods in a controlled temperature environment. This is because most of the drugs are temperature sensitive and require a desired temperature during storage in warehouses and during transportation.

10.2.6 DATA SECURITY

Security of data collected is also a major concern after analyzing the unfavorable features of centralized database as a threat to data security. Data gathered is also risky to put on a centralized database because of its less secured nature as compared to blockchain [12].

Following is the question asked here in this chapter:

Question: How to increase visibility and traceability in a medicine supply chain to solve the problems of drug shortages, counterfeiting, inventory management, and data security of cold chain shipping by using blockchain technology?

10.3   WHAT IS BLOCKCHAIN?

Blockchain technology is defined as the network of connected systems called blocks. Every block represents a piece of information. All systems connected to a blockchain are known as entities. All entities have a copy of every block with them, and whenever any person or system tries to edit data available in any block, it will reflect all entities in the network and access operation can't be performed without the verification process. Systems already present will check if the system that wants to make a transaction is an authorized person or not. After verification, approval for further processing will be given in this fashion and blockchain makes a network more secure by keeping eye on each transaction by every side. This is also known as Distributed Ledger Technology (DLT) [13,15,16]. This concept will be used for improving traceability in medicine supply chain and to close doors for counterfeiting of medicines.

10.4   PROPOSED SOLUTION

The proposed solution after accounting for major problems, challenges, and loopholes in the present system, along with blockchain as a major solution, makes use of IoT-enabled vehicles for cold shipping. IoT is the network of interrelated smart objects or devices that are able to collect data and exchange data over internet. In an IoT network, every object connected with every other object is called a "thing". These smart devices are embedded with sensors that are responsible for capturing data. Here in the proposed model/solution, IoT-enabled vehicles will be used for cold chain shipping purposes. They will ensure that the drug that needs to be transported between two entities in the supply chain will be getting desired controlled temperature to reach the destination in their original form. Whenever the temperature desired for the drug changes, sensor in the vehicle will automatically shift the temperature according to the need of a drug.

10.4.1 BLOCKCHAIN IN SUPPLY CHAIN

This solution talks about solving the issues of counterfeiting, inventory management, and data security of medicines by making use of blockchain technology for traceability and cold chain shipping with the help of transportation of medicines between different entities through IoT-enabled vehicles.

Entities in the blockchain which will have access to the information contained in blocks for keeping track of flow of medicines to avoid counterfeiting at any stage are classified as follows [5]:

1. Manufacturers
2. Distributors
3. Pharmacies (retailers and wholesalers)
4. Hospitals
5. Consumers
6. Travel agencies

First of all, a highly authorized body needs to be established which will work under the surveillance of government. The main function of this body is to assign a unique ID to the genuine and legitimate manufacturers and distributors present in the pharma industry and to regulate the movement of batches [14]. It will keep an eye on the functioning of manufacturers and distributors and will explain the uniform standards for their functioning.

The steps are as follows:

Step 1:

Manufacturers will be assigned a unique ID by the authorized body which will work as a private key for transaction between manufacturer and distributors. Manufacturing firm will send finished medicines to distributors according to the demand or order placed by them. This information will be added as a block in the blockchain network, and as a working mechanism of blockchain, all entities will be notified about this transaction. This block will contain the following information:

• Date of manufacturing
• Date of expiry
• Ingredients used and their composition
• Manufacturer's unique Id
• Manufacturing firm's name
• Date of dispatching

Step 2:
• Demanded batch of medicines will be transported to the distributor. For transportation, IoT-enabled vehicles will be used by transportation agencies for maintaining cold chain shipping. This will ensure that medicines will reach consumers in their original form as they will get desired controlled

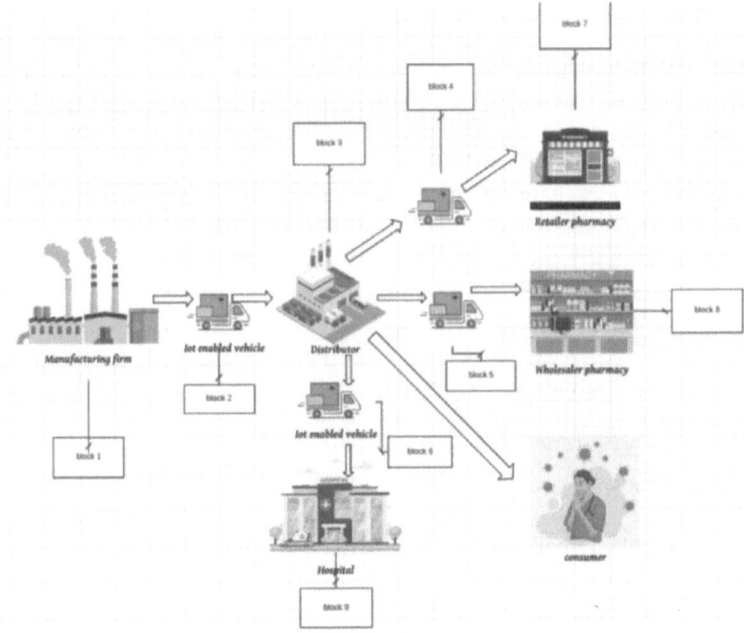

FIGURE 10.1 Drug flow from manufacturer to end users.

temperature with the help of IoT sensors embedded in the vehicle. This set of information will be added as a new block which will contain information, such as:

- Vehicle no.
- Travel agency's name (Figure 10.1).

Step 3:

Now distributor will receive the medicines with unique ID of manufacturer and other useful information. Here distributor's ID and manufacturer's ID will work as a private key between them. On receiving, arrival time will be noticed, and new information will be added by the distributor again through this transaction and all entities in the network will know that distributor has received the medicines.

New added information are as follows:

- Distributor's Id
- Arrival time
- Name of distributing firm
- Quantity of medicines

Step 4:

Here On completion of previous transaction by distributor on receiving the medicines from manufacturer, travel agency will also be notified as it is a part of blockchain network. So, they will take the drug from distributors to transfer them to hospitals, retailer pharmacies, and wholesaler pharmacies. This is the point where chances of counterfeiting are more. This transaction will also notify others so it fills the loophole in the supply chain. This block will contain:

- Travel agency's details
- Vehicle no.
- Dispatched time from distributor's warehouse

Step 5:

Drugs from distributors can be directly sent to hospitals and also to retailers and wholesale pharmacies. When drugs are directly sent to hospitals in this case, whole similar activity of addition of new block will take place with notification to all. This block will contain following info:

- Verification status
- Arrival time

Step 6:

If the distributor sends medicines to pharmacies, same procedure will repeat.

Consumer can get the medicine from retailer, now as being a part of blockchain network consumer will be aware of the source of medicine whether it is coming from an authorized source or not.

Proper tracking of information at every transaction in supply chain will help manufacturers to be aware of market demand, and they can manage inventory accordingly to answer the question of drug shortage. This traceability feature achieved by blockchain will also overcome the issue of counterfeiting.

Blockchain at the place of a centralized database will be used for storing data collected by IoT-enabled vehicles during transportation. Data collected by sensors embedded in vehicles used in transportation is a useful data for further processing, and sharing this data over a centralized database could be a data threat. As in a centralized database, all data and records are stored at a single location.

Consequently, it is easier for a malicious entity to make changes in the data as it is the only copy, but sometimes difficult to account for malicious entity and time-consuming. Whereas in blockchain system each entity will have (Figure 10.2 and 10.3).

A copy of all the information and no new transaction can take place without verification from any of the entity present in the network.

10.5 CONCLUSION

After a thorough study of the supply chain in pharmaceutical industry and knowing the different issues in the present system used by supply chains, this conclusion can be made that there are so many escape clauses in it which can lead to many major problems like drug shortage, counterfeiting of medicines, sensitive drug's transportation, and compromise that can directly affect a patient's health.

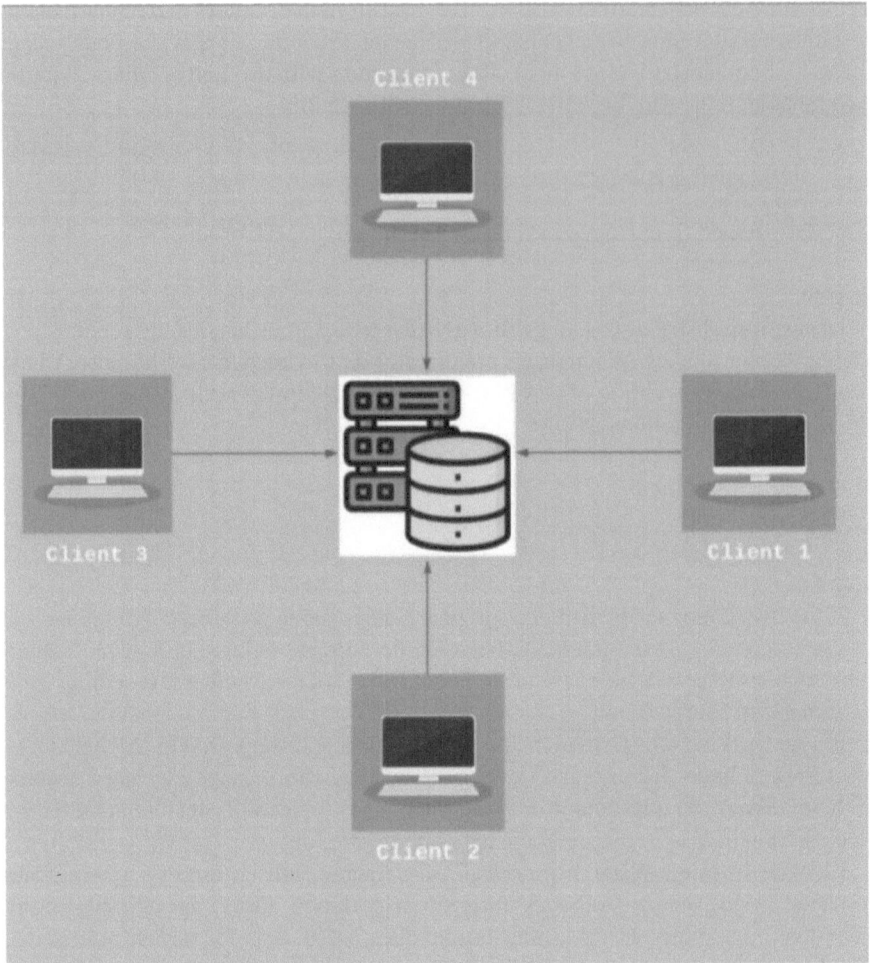

FIGURE 10.2 Centralized database.

As a solution to these major problems, blockchain technology can play a vital role in closing maximum escape clauses in the present system to improve visibility and traceability and to provide a clear far vision for the stakeholders present in pharmaceutical industry. This solution will not only improve the working efficiency of a medicine business cycle but also open gates for amazing opportunities for business in this sector. This blockchain solution could be used in the upcoming scenario of vaccine distribution of COVID-19 in India.

It will also result in fewer cases of deaths from falsified drugs and reduce suffering of patients due to drug shortage in the market.

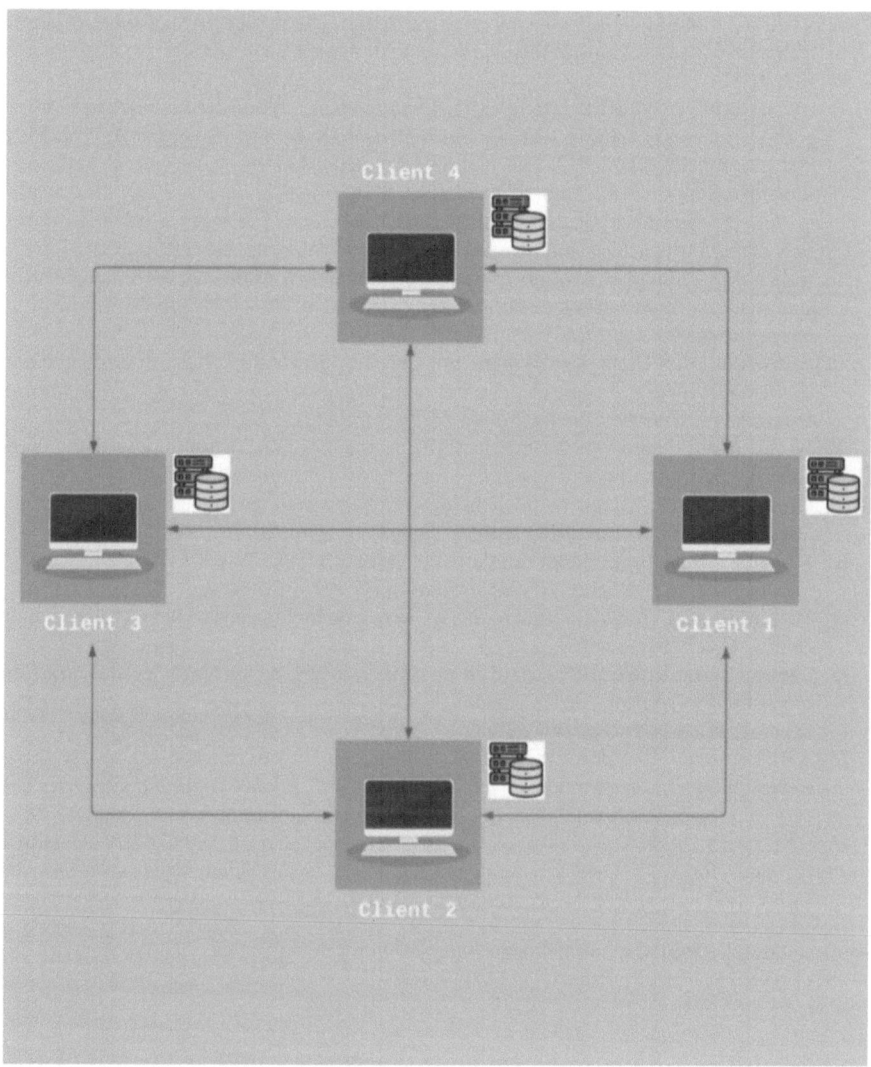

FIGURE 10.3 Blockchain Distributed system.

REFERENCES

1. Moulouki Reda, Dominique Kanga, Taif Fatima, Mohammed Azouazi, 2020. "Blockchain in health supply chain management: State of art challenges and opportunities", *Procedia Computer Science*, 175, 706–709.
2. Shashank Kumar, Ashok Kumar Pundir, 2020. "Blockchain, IoT enabled pharmaceutical supply chain for COVID-19", *5th NA International Conference on Industrial Engineering and Operations Management*, Michigan, USA.

3. Vladimir Plotnikov, Valentina Kuznetsova, 2018. "The prospects for the use of digital technology "Blockchain" in the pharmaceutical market", *MATEC Web of Conferences*, 193, 02029.
4. BW BUSINESSWORLD article, 2018. India in counterfeited medicines. https://www.google.com/amp/www.businessworld.in/amo/article/India-Emerges-As-Top-Five-Pharmaceuticals-Market-Of-The-World/05-05-2018-148349/.
5. Monalisa Sahoo, Sunil Samantha Singhar, Sony Snigdha Sahoo, 2020. "Blockchain model to eliminate drug counterfeiting", *Machine Learning and Information Processing, Advances in Intelligent Systems and Computing*, vol. 1101, pp. 213–224
6. Hala Awad, Zu'bi M.F. Al-Zu'bi, Al Zu'bi, Ayman Bahjat Abdallah, 2016. "Quantitative analysis of the causes of drug shortages in Jordan: A supply chain perspective", *International Business Research*, 9(6), 53–63.
7. Faisal Jamil, Lei Hang, KyuHyung Kim, Dohyeum Kim, 2019. "Anovel medical blockchain model for drug supply chain integrity management in a smart hospital", *Molecular Diversity Preservation International, Electronics*, 8(5).
8. World Health Organization Bulletin, 2010. Amount of false drugs in developing countries. https://www.who.int/bulletin/volumes/88/4/10-020410/en/.
9. Ijazul Haq, 2018. "Blockchain technology in pharmaceutical industry to prevent counterfeit drugs", *International Journal of Computer Applications*, 180(25), 93–305.
10. Mohammad Tamimi, Balan Sundarakani, Prakash Vel, 2010. "Cold chain logistics implementation strategies", *POMS Annual Conference, Canada*.
11. Yezhuvath Vinesh Balakrishnan, 2019. "Blockchain for robust and efficient supply chain", A TCS white paper.
12. Leeway hertz article. Blockchain in pharma industry. https://www.leewayhertz.com/blockchain-in-pharma-supply-chain/.
13. R3 blog, What is blockchain technology. https://www.r3.com/blockchain-101/.
14. S.R. Bryatov, A.A. Borodinov, 2019. "Blockchain in pharmaceutical supply chain: Researching a business model on hyper ledger fabric", *5th International Conference on Information Technology and Nanotechnology,* Samara, Russia.
15. S.M. Idrees, M. Nowostawski, R. Jameel, 2021. Blockchain-based digital contact tracing apps for COVID-19 pandemic management: Issues, challenges, solutions, and future directions. *JMIR Medical Informatics*, 9(2), e25245.
16. Idrees, S.M., Nowostawski, M., Jameel, R., Mourya, A.K., 2021. Security Aspects of Blockchain Technology Intended for Industrial Applications. Electronics 2021, 10, 951. https://doi.org/10.3390/electronics10080951

11 Sustainable and Effective Blockchain-based Solutions for the Security and Privacy of Healthcare Data

Sana Zeba and Mohammad Amjad
Jamia Millia Islamia

CONTENTS

11.1 INTRODUCTION

In the current era, the next frontier in the medical healthcare system is blockchain technology. The quick growth of modern healthcare systems used actuators and sensors devices for operating and monitoring the patient's health from time to time. Smart healthcare systems are an illustration of innovative smart and rapid growth wireless systems which exploit sensing, actuating, smart computing, artificial

DOI: 10.1201/9781003141471-11

intelligence, emerging blockchain technology, and networking technologies for checking patients remotely as well as maintaining health records of patients in digital form. These terms aim to enhance the surveillance of diseases and their causes, the management of drugs, the superiority of medical services and medicines, and the development of global strategies for chronic disease prevention. In 2009, the U.S. has attempted to conventional health agencies to implement Electronic Health Record (EHR) programs to track their patient healthcare and program data rather than position traditional paper approaches, the Health Information Technology for Economic and Clinical Health Act (HITECH) committed to approximately $36.5 billion (Al Omar et al., 2017). The original paper-based health reports for patients have now switched to electronic health records (EHRs) (Chakraborty et al., 2019). The electronic health record (EHR) market is currently valued at tens of billions of dollars, and various companies have transferred capital into the development of commercial EHRs and other wireless health data management systems-related healthcare applications.

The growth and evaluation of the healthcare system increased the security challenges, the privacy problems, and the leakage of the integrity of the system since its wireless connectivity and openly accessing damage the security of the system. In the smart healthcare system, adjustment of security and privacy has represented substantial threats for both hospitals or clinics and patients as well. To address the security and privacy problems and situations, there is a need for researchers to propose many solutions which are focused on these challenges of the modern healthcare system. Emerging and efficient blockchain technology may offer pervasive and sustainable solutions to smart healthcare systems which have the biggest security and privacy challenges.

A variety of new innovative application opportunities have been created by the disruptive and evolving study boom in blockchain technology, including smart transport, smart environment, smart world, and smart healthcare system applications.

The smart electronic healthcare system requires much consideration to the security, privacy, accuracy, and authenticity of the patient health data stored in the electronic healthcare record (EHR) and also has been a prerequisite that patient's health data must be managed in a proper mode. Hence, for managing the access of EHR and storage of the patient's electronic health data to monitor and manage the transactions, we tend to suggest the thought of blockchain technology which has a decentralized association of several shareholders such as doctors, patients, pharmacy, hospital, test lab, imaging centers, pathology, and insurance organizations.

As an example, a remote patient monitoring system (RPM) has provided the management and monitoring of patient's health outside of traditional clinics and hospitals. Firstly, it permits patients the convenience of healthcare service. The patients can easily stay connected remotely with healthcare providers when required. It also diminishes healthcare costs and medical access time and enhances the quality of patient care. But there is also a lack of security in the health remote patient monitoring (RPM) system because of its open, wireless connectivity.

In the present situations, blockchain technology is the greatest pervasive, emerging, sustainable, and growing technology in the security and data privacy area of

Alt Text of Chapter Images

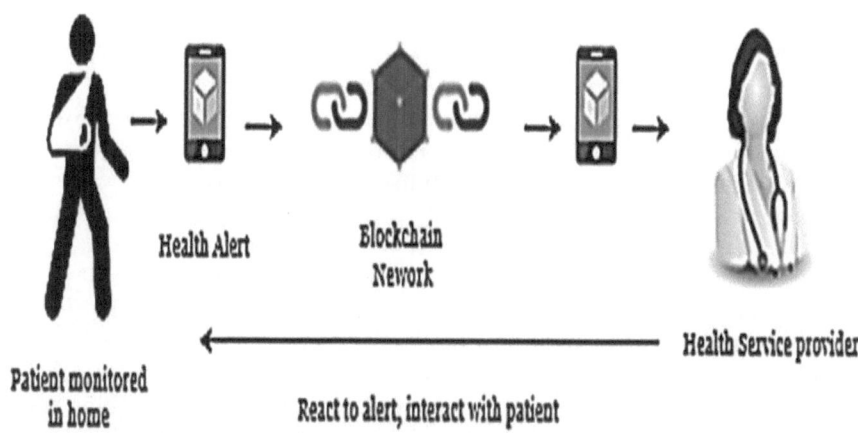

FIGURE 11.1   Patient monitoring remotely (Dwivedi et al., 2019).

healthcare systems and its applications, because of its features like peer-to-peer, distributed, decentralized storage, smart contracts, immutable ledgers, and cryptography. The remote patient monitoring (RPM) system has provided in a secure manner blockchain technology for healthcare organizations to handle and protect the patient's data and prevent the alteration or modification of patient information while maintaining its accuracy. This patient monitoring system used the blockchain network to handle any transaction among the patients and healthcare service providers. The blockchain network of the RPM system makes it decentralized, distributed, and more secure (Figure 11.1).

This chapter discusses the growing need for uniform levels of protection of data in smart healthcare computing systems, and our major goal is to perform a systematic review with summarized existing problems of smart healthcare systems and provide solutions related to the securities and privacy of its data with the blockchain technology. Then, the detailed technical concepts that may be applied to enhance security and privacy in healthcare systems at both levels like organization and patient levels are considered.

The outline of this chapter is as follows: Section 11.2 discusses the electronic health records and cloud-based healthcare system, Section 11.3 shows the security concern in the conventional healthcare system and privacy of patient's data, Section 11.4 explains blockchain overview, blockchain technology in the healthcare system, features of blockchain, types of blockchain, consensus mechanism in blockchain, smart contracts, and applications of blockchain in health data systems, Section 11.5 gives the literature review study, Section 11.6 gives sustainable and pervasive computing paradigm for the healthcare system, Section 11.7 concludes the chapter, and the last section discusses some future work in the healthcare system.

11.2 ELECTRONIC HEALTH RECORDS
AND CLOUD-BASED HEALTHCARE SYSTEM

Mostly, electronic medical records (EMRs) or electronic health records (EHR) contain the health and clinical data of the patients and are stored by correspondent healthcare service providers. This electronic record enables the retrieval and investigation of patient's healthcare data. Firstly, designed the Health Information Systems (HIS) which create new HER instances and store them. HIS are normally the front-end of a database at the back-end, in a centralized manner or distributed way implementation. Healthcare systems become interoperable among patients and different healthcare service providers through EMR solutions.

For example, electronic medical records (EMRs) are planned to permit patient medical history to exchange with the patient or be made available to multiple healthcare service providers like from a rustic hospital to a capital city hospital of the country. Newly, the pervasiveness of various smart devices like android devices, iOS devices, and wearable devices has also caused a paradigm shift within smart healthcare companies. All these smart devices can be user-owned or they can be installed by the healthcare service provider to monitor the well-being of the patients and update/facilitate medical health treatment and measuring of patients.

For example, there is a wide variety of mobile applications related to health, increase height, fitness, weight loss, and other categories related to healthcare. These applications mainly operate as a management tool, tracking tool, for registering patient's fitness exercises or workouts and keeping the records of consumed calories and so on. There are also various smart devices embedded with sensors to measure heartbeat, also measure during a workout, or other devices for self-testing of the sugar level. For example, Leu and collaborators projected a wireless body sensor based on a smartphone to collect a user or patient's physiological data using this body sensor which is embedded in a smart shirt (Esposito et al., 2018).

The data can be constantly obtained and sent to a mobile computer in real time for monitoring, before being sent for further processing to the healthcare cloud. A further example in healthcare is Ambient Assisted Living resolutions and healthcare systems that provide remote personal health supervision for automated telemedicine and telehealth programs. Personal health records (PHR) used smart mobile or smart wearable devices for monitoring and collecting patient's health data (Figure 11.2).

However, there are several issues related to personal health records, because of the ability to support real-time health data accessing and sharing of cloud computing, which has used in remote personal healthcare records. Figure 11.2 demonstrates how to use cloud computing for sharing and accessing healthcare data among service providers, various departments of health care, and providing a way of swapping and possibly certifying patient's data between EMR or EHR and PHR. Hence, it generates a comprehensive view of the health medical records of every patient.

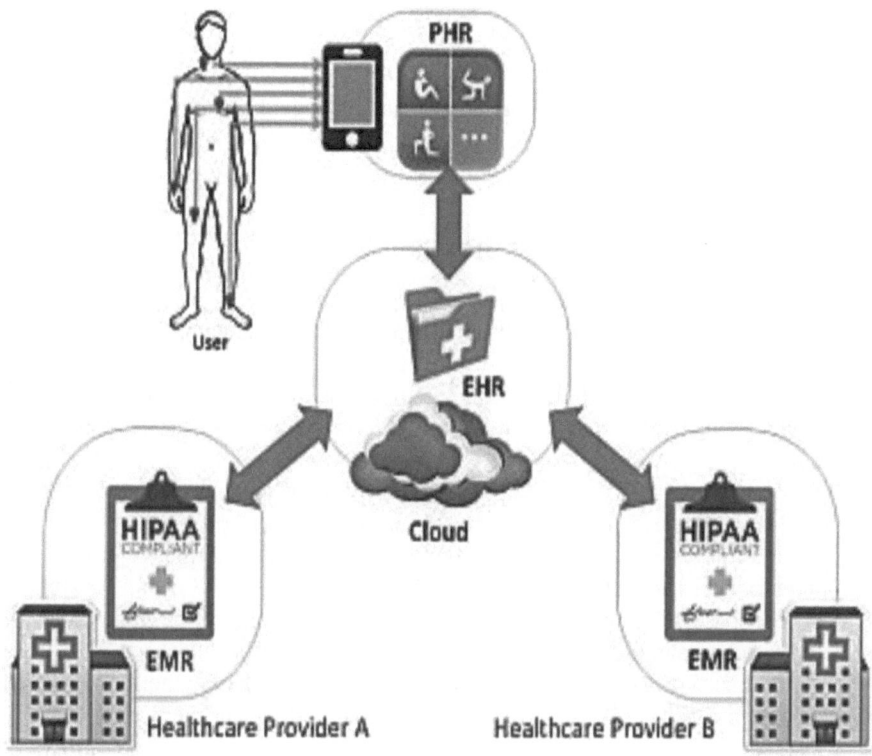

FIGURE 11.2   Conventional cloud-based electronic healthcare system (Esposito et al., 2018).

11.3   SECURITY CONCERN IN CONVENTIONAL HEALTHCARE SYSTEM

In this era, security is the prime concern in any wireless applications like medical healthcare system, smart world IoT system, smart home system, and smart transportation. There has been increasing courtesy in mobile health data, disjointed electronic healthcare records (EHR), and connected different departments of healthcare data applications for improving security and accuracy of patient medicine. While it has also provided better access and shared control of patient's In cloud computing-based healthcare environments, there are different challenges and limitations to using conventional cryptographic primitives and health management control systems to discourse security and privacy majors. The traditional cloud computing-based centralized healthcare systems struggle because of their centralized nature. There are so many problems faced in the healthcare system like medical data privacy, single point of failure, and healthcare system vulnerability.

We shortly mention some required properties of the healthcare system related to security and privacy below.

- **Pseudonymity:** No user will be able to find any healthcare system part and any department of the system.
- **Privacy:** Only registered departments will be able to interrelate with the healthcare system.
- **Integrity:** Only authenticated departments will be able to handle the private data.
- **Accountability:** Different departments will hold their separate block-id, and that id no users will be able to interrelate with that actual department of the block.
- **Security:** Encrypted health data will be kept by the departments in the system which enhances an additional level of security in the healthcare system.
- **Confidentiality:** Confidentiality of health data means protecting the patient's private information from leaks to unauthorized providers.
- **Availability:** Availability of data refers to that patient's information is available for accessing and sharing when it is needed.
- **Authenticity:** Private sensitive data of patients should not be updated or accessed by any unauthorized users.
- **Authorization:** Authorization in healthcare records refers to the procedure of permitting to patients, services providers, or different medical departments for doing anything.

The new conventional consolidated electronic medical record (EMR) or electronic health record (EHR) systems are responsible for malicious attacks such as Denial Service, Black Hole attacks, and DDoS attacks. Furthermore, we are researching the likely use of blockchain technologies to sustain stable cloud-hosted healthcare records.

11.3.1 Privacy of Patient Data

In the U.S., guidelines on patient healthcare records are governed by the Health Insurance Portability and Accountability Act of 1996 (HIPAA) (Qiu et al., 2018). Privacy and integrity of health data require more concern because of the open and centralized nature of healthcare networks. The HIPAA act guarantees the protection, accuracy, and privacy of the health data of entities, although still allowing the movement of medical health data necessary for the well-organized administration of health service providers (Zaghloul et al., 2019).

Hence, the blockchain technology-based network used follows the principle of complete privacy and secrecy on the patient identification associated with a particular transaction. Subsequently, at the time of its beginning, blockchain technology has felt a research that has verified several kinds of methods to sort out the problem of the conventional healthcare access control system.

11.4 BLOCKCHAIN OVERVIEW

Blockchain technology concept acts as a database that is used for the storage of data in the network in a decentralized manner (Idrees et al., 2021). It is an immutable record of network transactions stored in a distributed ledger which are distributed among the departments to confirm decentralized and secure transactions. It is an arrangement of blocks, and all blocks are linked to the chain. Every chain has one parent block, and every first block of the chain is called a genesis block, and there is no parent block for the genesis block.

Blockchain technology has the concept of the peer-to-peer and distributed ledger. This public distributed ledger has three notions like block, chain, and transaction. In the blockchain, a block is the storage part to store the transactions, hash values, and data. The chain is the connecting part of blockchain which is used for joining the blocks and creating chains. Any valuable info which is scattered in the network of various applications is called the transactions (Figure 11.3).

There are so many definitions of blockchain based on its valuable features and operating nature. Some definitions of blockchain are as follows:

i. **Blockchain as Data Structure:** The blockchain mentions a kind of data structure that allows identifying and tracking digital transactions and sharing this transaction information across the distributed network of devices, to create a distributed trust network.

ii. **Blockchain as Database:** The blockchain has been defined as a back-end database that sustains a distributed ledger that can be examined openly.

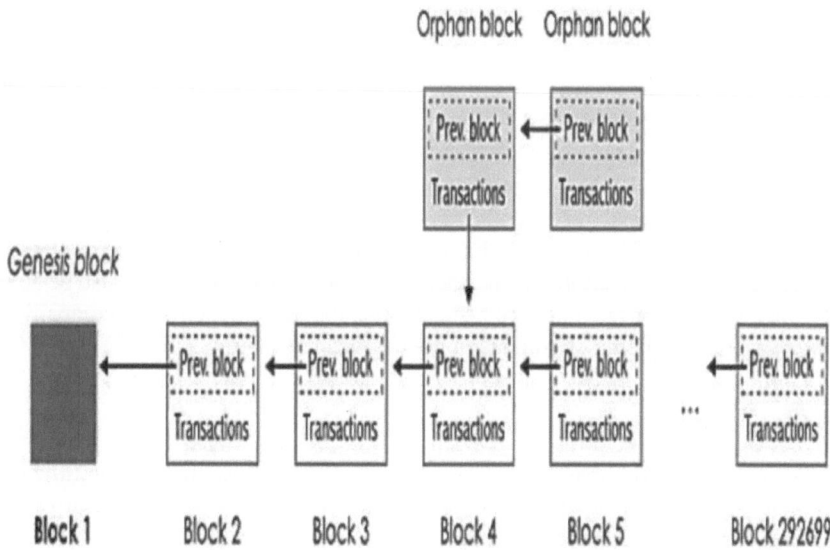

FIGURE 11.3 Blockchain example.

   iii. **Blockchain as Distributed Ledger:** The blockchain is a public distributed
        ledger that is replicated across several devices gathered in a peer-to-peer
        distributed network.
   iv. **Blockchain Business Definition:** The blockchain acts as an exchange net-
        work for moving digital transactions, assets, and value, among peers, with-
        out the support of any intermediaries.

11.4.1 BLOCKCHAIN TECHNOLOGY IN HEALTHCARE SYSTEM

The decentralized blockchain technology can be employed to alleviate the risks facing by electronic healthcare systems. The decentralized behavior of blockchain allows
it to improve transparency because it cannot be manipulated by any third party or
possessors of health care. The blockchain-based healthcare system will enable medical users to secure the money transaction during medical treatment. This technology
has vigorous encryption of health data that is capable of maintaining the security of
patient's sensitive information and making it visible to the different authorized departments in the healthcare system. Thus, the sensitive payment transaction information is
secured from cybercriminals who steal sensitive evidence from the electronic healthcare patient's data and customers as well as other healthcare applications.

  Blockchain technology in health care may eradicate hazards of patient experience
when they access or store their medical health information on their android or iOS
smartphone. Smart mobiles are prone to attackers who access their mobile health-
related information without any agreement with patients. However, blockchain-based
healthcare systems provide storage capability to user where their medical sensitive
info will be safe from third providers of health care. The health data are stored
in a locked manner because of the data encryption and decryption in the system.
Furthermore, the blockchain transparent manner allows the authority to manage the
patients as well as the various departments of the system. Hence, the only authorized
users (e.g., patients) are the members who have been permitted to access or share the
health data stored in the database of the system.

  Electronic healthcare record (EHR) systems are vulnerable to security and privacy concerns. Blockchain technology may have countless benefits to support the
healthcare security and privacy of the patient's data and the operations of healthcare organizations. The secure technology will improve the medicine development
of the healthcare association. Furthermore, the healthcare records will also be able to
minimize the fake drugs that have been an obligation to the medicinal company that
interprets poor medicine of patients in the healthcare system.

11.4.2 FEATURES OF BLOCKCHAIN

Blockchain technology has the characteristics of interoperability, decentralization,
immutability, anonymity, etc. which merge with the electronic healthcare record
(HER or EMR) system and become a secure blockchain-based digital healthcare
system. All the nodes (e.g., service providers) work in coordination, and all providers
can join, rejoin, and even leave the network. So, here we can merge all the features
of blockchain as follows:

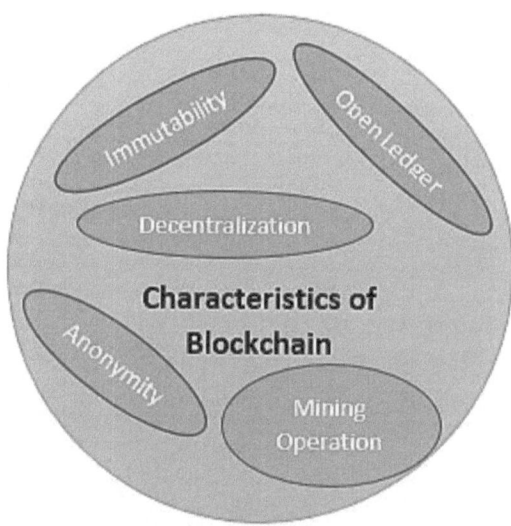

FIGURE 11.4   Features of blockchain.

- **Decentralization:** It is the prime characteristic of blockchain technology in that it does not trust centralized nodes (e.g., departments).
- **Transparent:** All the health data which are stored in chain forms are secured and transparent to all the nodes (e.g., providers).
- **Open-Source:** Blockchain can be easily accessible to anybody to create any security applications (Figure 11.4).
- **Autonomous:** Every block of blockchain can update or transfer independently its data securely, and it maintains trust between departments.
- **Immutability:** Since data in blockchain will be kept forever and cannot be altered or changed.
- **Peer-to-Peer Network:** Blockchain technology removes systems central dependencies of all providers from any central department within the network.
- **Distributed and Open Ledger:** Each provider of the health care in the network validated separately and acted as transparent in the healthcare organization.
- **Mining Operation:** In healthcare applications, the mining operation of blockchain adds medical-related transactions in the public ledger of a previous transaction.

11.4.3   Types of Blockchain

The blockchain is classified into different types based on access controlling power of the medical-related network. There are four types of blockchain, which are as follows:

1. **Public Blockchain:** For openly accessing the healthcare records, we used the public blockchain because there is no restriction in the public blockchain-based healthcare network. Public healthcare organizations used

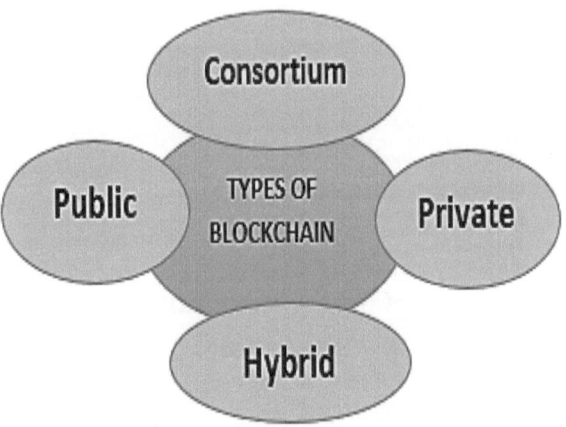

FIGURE 11.5   Types of blockchain.

mostly Proof of Work as the consensus algorithms while the Proof of Stake (PoS) and DPoS also come under this blockchain. Examples of this block-chain are Bitcoin, Ethereum, Monero, Litecoin, Dash, etc.

2. **Private Blockchain:** The private blockchain-based applications have restrictions for accessing the applications. Any node (e.g., providers or departments) cannot join the private network unless administrators invited it. Private blockchain used consensus algorithms which are RAFT, the Practical Byzantine fault tolerance (PBFT), etc. Examples of the private blockchain are Multichain, MONAX.

3. **Consortium or Federated Blockchain:** The consortium blockchain used the semi-decentralized concept. This type of healthcare application is con-trolled and constrained by more than one organization of applications. This kind of blockchain is mainly used by government applications like banks. Examples of consortium blockchain are Corda, B3i (insurance), EWF (energy), and R3 (bank).

4. **Hybrid Blockchain:** This blockchain is the combination of both the pub-lic and the private blockchain. This hybrid blockchain used the features or characteristics of both blockchain (Figure 11.5).

11.4.4   CONSENSUS MECHANISM IN BLOCKCHAIN

Blockchains communicate trust by making each node (e.g., providers) handle their blockchain copy on the medical network, but have their ledger copy for each node (e.g., providers) and enable a distributed process to approve the existing state of the blockchain. This distributed process is recognized and defined as the algorithm that creates the basis for anonymity, protection, transparency, and dependence on a block-chain as a consensus protocol. The consensus algorithm must validate the sequence of transactions and outcomes of smart contract executions. There are many suggested and diverse types of consensus protocols, but only a few of them are very common. Below are several consensus protocols mentioned.

1) **Proof of Work (PoW):** Undoubtedly, Proof of Work (PoW) is the highest consensus protocol. PoW is often used in the public network as it helps anyone to join the blockchain authentication blocks. So-called miners are needed to overcome a cryptographic "puzzle" calculation while verifying a new block with the brute force approach, the miners attempt to find a hash value of the new block with a value lower than the already determined block value. The miners get awarded who computes this hash value firstly and validates the transactions. A main weakness of the PoW protocol is, it demands high energy as well as high computing time when this consensus protocol is applied on a large blockchain.

2) **Proof of Stake (PoS):** The selection of an approved node is identified with the stake value of each node in the blockchain. However, this might be giving a partial benefit to the "richest" node because the node having the most balance has more chances to participate. Therefore, there is a drawback for the node having the lowest balance. To justify this, numerous hybrid forms of PoS have been recommended where the stake value is combined with some randomization for the selection of the approved node. The largest cryptocurrency Ethereum is preparing to move from PoW to PoS.

3) **Practical Byzantine Fault Tolerance (PBFT):** For those events that require faster transaction computation times, or cannot manage the cost of PoW consensus, one substitute is Practical Byzantine Fault Tolerance (PBFT) (Hardin & Kotz, 2019). Byzantine agreement protocol concepts are used in Practical Byzantine Fault Tolerance (Hasselgren et al., 2020). Three phases can be well-defined in the PBFT consensus protocol:
   i)   pre-prepared,
   ii) prepared, and
   iii) commit

Each node in the network wants two-thirds of the votes to move through these three phases. Because of the multicast messages of this consensus, it does not impose high computational expenses. For this reason, the best use of PBFT is in a consortium blockchain, which has a minor group of semi-trusted organizations. Currently, PBFT is used in Hyperledger Fabric.

11.4.5 SMART CONTRACTS

Some blockchain infrastructures support smart contracts. These are computer functions or self-executing contractual agreements that are stored on the blockchain infrastructure. Smart contracts can be called explicitly by users or set up to trigger on some event. When smart-contract programs are called, and then, each node in the network executes the source code and verifies the result against other nodes through the consensus protocol. The smart function call can be appended onto the blockchain, as a transaction, for verification purposes. It is significant to note, still, that smart contract code cannot be modified after it is added in blockchain due to immutability property.

Subsequently, smart contracts are automatically imposed based on these pre-agreed provisions, and all nodes work without the contribution of any third party or intermediate. This operation with smart contracts can be awoken in a transaction, and the use of this blockchain functionality appears to be tempting to the healthcare application.

11.4.6 Applications of Blockchain in Health Data Systems

In recent years, blockchain has a wide range of optimum reliability applications and uses in healthcare systems such as Smart Healthcare Management System, Smart Home, Smart Banking System, and Online Information Storage Management System. The distributed ledger technology helps the secure transfer of health records of the patient and the medicine supply chain management. Blockchain technology can renovate healthcare records, placing the patients at the center of the ecosystem and enhancing the privacy, security, and interoperability of medical health-related data. This decentralized technology could offer a new infrastructure for health information exchanges (HIE) by creating electronic medical records or electronic health records (EMR/EHR) more efficient, well-organized, disintermediated, and secure.

For professionals and patients, blockchain and healthcare organizations are presently working on or have released blockchain-based healthcare systems to enhance health care. Blockchain technology has become a valuable tool for healthcare records, transforming the healthcare industry worldwide because of decentralizing medical history of patients, tracking pharmaceuticals, and refining the medical payment options. Some blockchain applications in health care are discussed below:

- For improving medical record access of health record access
- For reducing costs in health care
- For improving electronic medical record
- For stopping counterfeit medicines
- For tracking clinical tests and pharmaceuticals
- For tracking medical credentials
- For enhancing the security and privacy of healthcare-related transactions
- For improving patient-doctor interactions
- For preventing diseases.

11.5 LITERATURE REVIEW

Hardin and Kotz (2019), has presented a deployment related to blockchain implementations in healthcare data structures, that has been designed in their work. The authors addressed some of the security problems, privacy, and concert trade-offs, related to the use of blockchain in data networks for health care. Finding the health data analysis that focused on blockchain technologies to put greater emphasis on real-world implementations and monitoring, smart contract stability, efficient and accessible inspection tools, blockchain regulation, and adherence to rules and standards for the health data framework.

Leila Ismail et al. (2019) has proposed healthcare data management architecture with a lightweight blockchain that decreases the communication and computational overhead compared to the Bitcoin network by isolating the network contestants into clusters and also maintaining one copy of the ledger per cluster. Besides, the author has suggested an interpretation that is dominant in the Bitcoin network to discourage forking. A HBCM that produces the blocks and orders the transactions is used in the proposed architecture. They have also analyzed the effectiveness of the proposed architecture in providing security and privacy by examining the different threats of the Bitcoin network.

Seyednima Khezr et al. (2019) have discussed a comprehensive review of emergent blockchain-based healthcare data and related health applications and called attention to the open research matters in healthcare The author has offered an IoMT application of blockchain which generates data endlessly. Also, discussed the main problem of the healthcare data system that requires consideration from researchers is how the blockchain technology will operate in incomposite and diverse communication systems.

Ashutosh Dhar Dwivedi et al. (2019) have proposed a novel hybrid framework with modified blockchain technology models appropriate to IoT devices that trust on their decentralized distributed nature and other supplementary security and privacy assets of the network. In this paper, the author combines the rewards of the public key, private key, advanced lightweight cryptographic scheme, and blockchain technology to develop the patient-centric remotely access control system. The solutions of the healthcare system given here make healthcare data and transactions more secure and unspecified over a blockchain-based decentralized network. In the future, the researchers can implement the system in a testable system to offer some real work security assurances.

Jinglin Qiu et al. (2018) have discussed the integration of the healthcare system with blockchain concept and also exposed the healthcare industry to security and privacy challenges which include patients' healthcare data privacy and security of mobile healthcare users in the vicinity. The main motivation of using blockchain in healthcare systems is to solve the data integrity, interoperability of data, and privacy issues in recent remote healthcare systems. This covers the way for future research work on the development of smart healthcare systems.

Anton Hasselgrena et al. (2020) has been designed a systematically review, and synthesize peer-reviewed, to utilized blockchain services for recovering the healthcare system and organization of health education. The boundary of research in this review has to show that blockchain-based resolutions presently are being explored in a few clinical pilot system use cases. The main purpose of this paper was how to use blockchain for protecting healthcare patients' data.

Ehab Zaghloul et al. (2019) have proposed a novel scheme to share and manage data schemes that permit patients over their health records by leveraging the privacy issue and security benefits of blockchain and smart contracts. In this paper, the authors also compare current methods for healthcare data management with proposed schemes and conclude that they permit patients over their health data and reduce the dependencies on data generated through healthcare organizations. Additionally, they presented a secure and private medical health record sharing and management scheme. They show the security and privacy analysis of patients that can protect against credible threats to securely and privately share their data with blockchain. Blockchain and smart contracts show that patients can share their health records in a secure manner that preserves the desired privacy. In the future, the author has planned on validating the proposed scheme and security analysis.

Sabyasachi Chakraborty et al. (2019) have proposed a methodology to describe in the work fully overcomes the problem in terms of efficiency and also reduces the problem of the security and privacy of the patient data that is being generated in the conventional healthcare data system. The proposed framework has well established the complete supervision of a treatment or an ongoing cure or generic healthcare from the starting to the very end. The framework uses the consensus of multiple stakeholders to ensure the authenticity of generated data, and after that, it is stored and has been combined to the chain of blockchain.

Arijit Saha et al. (2019) have offered the state-of-the-art blockchain-based medical healthcare systems of health organizations. In this paper, the author has discussed numerous existing works of a similar arena and also offered a comparative study among the earlier published works related to the healthcare system with blockchain. There has reviewed of all possible research works on medical healthcare using blockchain technology with a suitable comparative study. Still, the same paper also highlights security and privacy issues on the blockchain-based medical healthcare system.

Vidhya Ramani et al. (2018) have proposed a secure and efficient blockchain-based data accessibility approach for the patients and the specialist of the correspondent healthcare data system. Hence, this paper considered blockchain technology as a decentralized distributed mechanism to protect the patient data in healthcare systems. The proposed system can defend the privacy and security of the patients as well. Still, they analyzed that the proposed scheme can attain the requirements of integrity, confidentiality, and authentication. Also, there has been proposed a possible smart contract agreement for considering this healthcare scenario.

Abdullah Al Omar et al. (2017) have offered a secure and privacy anxiety healthcare data management system with blockchain technology for the storage of patient's health data. The core idea of this research work is to reserve the delicate healthcare data on the blockchain to achieve privacy, accountability, integrity, and security. This paper represents a privacy-preserving mechanism for the patient's healthcare data. With the investigation of the protocol, the author has shown the strengths of the developed platform of the healthcare system. The complete purpose of this paper is to develop a decentralized distributed healthcare system and divert the healthcare web platform in a distributed way for the patients.

Swathi et al. (2019) have created a system with public and private keys using the Elliptic-Curve cryptography that allows users to create wallets. The proposed healthcare blockchain of this paper has the potential to involve millions of individuals, patients, healthcare organization providers, healthcare entities, and medical field researchers to share the massive amount of diet, genetic, lifestyle, environmental, and healthcare data with a guaranteed security solution and privacy protection. Blockchain technology absolutely has a place in the healthcare IT ecosystem, and the ONC should powerfully consider basing their interoperability property and also use blockchain decentralized nature.

11.6   SUSTAINABLE AND PERVASIVE COMPUTING PARADIGM

The revolutionary blockchain technology behind the Bitcoin cryptocurrency, which is secured, interoperable and decentralized, hence, it can act as the liberator for the healthcare Internet of Things (IoT) applications security. The field of smart healthcare systems has been a growing use of medical sensors for monitoring remote and real-time health records with the outline of sustainable computing paradigm like the Internet of Things (IoT). The sustainable paradigm demonstrated is a healthcare IoT system that demands the use of the IoT module to capture and fetch the medical data that have been generated by the patient's wearable device. Preferably, the blockchain is utilized for storing and maintaining the medical data of the users in the form of several transactions. The machine learning concept is used for detecting anomalies and certain scenarios that may get up for basic identification of the health conditions that are tackled by the patients.

Still, the medical sensors create and process a massive amount of personal health data related to a patient's condition that needs to be secured from any cyberattacks. We create a sustainable blockchain computing paradigm for patients storing their health-related information like disease, health insurance, doctor, lab test results, and medicine in the electronic health record (EHR) forms. If patients take appointment in different hospitals, then patients are identified through previous digital details using the patient key.

But in the situation of remote healthcare application, the major concern arises in the order to security and privacy of the patient's data because of its interoperability of several stakeholders' providers in the healthcare process. Therefore, the concern of privacy and security also mitigation of the precise health data has been controlled in the paradigm by regulating, sensing, and monitoring sustainable paradigm with an agreement to the healthcare IoT and the blockchain as a transaction for placing out trusted and accurate data for serving with cautious medical healthcare and profits to the patients across the world (Figure 11.6).

With the rapid growth in electronic health records (EHR) or electronic medical records (EMR), cloud health data storage, and new security protection regulations, innovative opportunities are opening for healthcare organizations, as well as provide secure access and share patient's healthcare records. Figure 11.6 demonstrates five steps of the healthcare record management roadmap in blockchain, which are discussed below. Blockchain-based healthcare applications include data sharing, data storage on the cloud, data management, and EMR or EHR, which are explained in detail below.

Step-1: Primary raw data are created by the communication between patient, doctors, and specialists. This record consists of health history, present problems, and other information related to physiology.

Step-2: An EHR or EMR is generated for each patient using the collected primary raw data of the first step. Other medical info such as nursing care, medical tests, and drug history and MRI information are also included in EMR or EHR.

Step-3: Specific patients who have the rights to sensitive EMR records, and customized access control is granted only to the proprietor of this property.

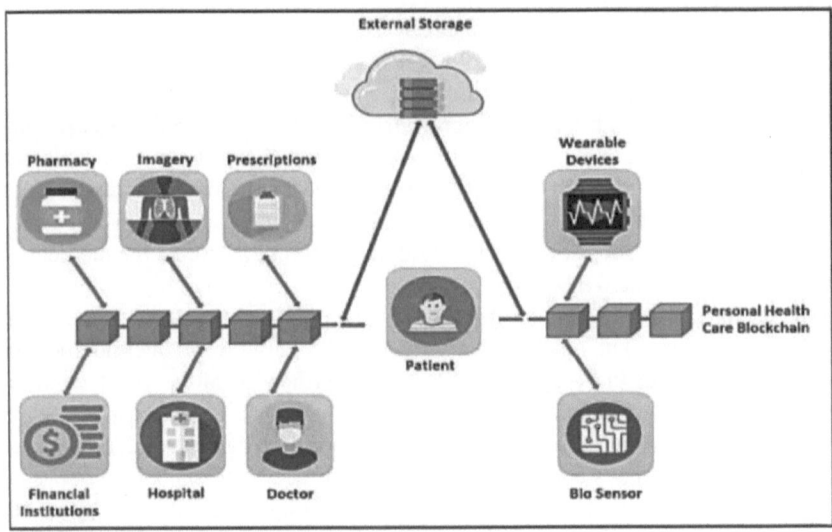

FIGURE 11.6   Complete blockchain-based healthcare system (Chakraborty et al., 2019).

Providers or departments who need to access such appreciated info must appeal permission which is forwarded to the owner of EHR, and then, the owner will decide to whom access will be approved.

Step-4: This step is the core part of the complete process of healthcare management including database, the blockchain network, and cloud-based storage. Data are stored in a distributed manner with database and cloud storage, and blockchain technology provides extreme security and privacy to ensure authentic access and sharing of medical records.

Step-5: Healthcare service providers such as ad hoc ambulatory or clinic, community healthcare center, and hospitals are the end operator who desires to get access and share for a safe delivery which will be approved by the owner. For example, no matter where you are, your health or medical record will be presented and accessible on your mobile and validated through a public distributed ledger such as blockchain, to which healthcare service providers would continue to merge over time.

11.7   CONCLUSION

The current study gave an overview of a pervasive and sustainable computing paradigm for the security-related concern in healthcare management systems as well as the applications of blockchain technology in the healthcare application. In fact, because of the rapid growth of this paradigm, blockchain has been used in numerous use cases of health care and medicine to improve the automated medical services for the users.

To make this perilous healthcare information more secure and locked, there has been a need to use blockchain technology. Our review shows that the mainly researches focusing blockchain for enhancing the security of healthcare toward sharing and accessing electronic medical records or electronic health records. Other surveys should be measured by blockchain researchers in the field like insurance service, biomedical research, and pharmaceutical supply chain.

Still, blockchain offers auspicious features, even though there is a requirement for more exploration to better knowledge to develop and estimate this technology. Constant efforts have been shown to reduce limitations in scalability, privacy, and security to improve service providers' confidence to use this technology and to increase its adoption in the applications of healthcare systems.

11.8   FUTURE WORK

While blockchain's integrity and digital storage design offer electronic healthcare data management possibilities, these features also include several challenges that are important for further research. The data integrity feature of blockchain technologies results in immutability, which ensures that all information will not be erased or changed until stored. But if the record includes health data, this kind of private data would fall under the defense of privacy law, and all of them would not allow private data to be indefinitely reserved, Article 17 of the General Data Protection Regulation.

Another real-world challenge is how appropriate it is for the blockchain to store medical health records. Initially, blockchain was developed to store transaction data that are comparatively limited in size and linear. However, healthcare data such as test results and medication schedules may be broad and relational, taking further research. It is considered to be the most secured data. At the same time, permanent medical data hash values are kept on-chain in the blockchain to validate the safety, reliability, and consistency of off-chain health information. Such understanding will mitigate future difficulties.

REFERENCES

Al Omar, A., Rahman, M.S., Basu, A., & Kiyomoto, S. (2017). Medibchain: A blockchain based privacy preserving platform for healthcare data. *International Conference on Security, Privacy and Anonymity in Computation, Communication and Storage*, Guangzhou, China, pp. 534–543.

Chakraborty, S., Aich, S., & Kim, H.-C. (2019). A secure healthcare system design framework using blockchain technology. *2019 21st International Conference on Advanced Communication Technology (ICACT)*, PyeongChang, Korea, pp. 260–264.

Dwivedi, A.D., Srivastava, G., Dhar, S., & Singh, R. (2019). A decentralized privacy-preserving healthcare blockchain for IoT. *Sensors, 19*(2), 326.

Esposito, C., De Santis, A., Tortora, G., Chang, H., & Choo, K.-K.R. (2018). Blockchain: A panacea for healthcare cloud-based data security and privacy? *IEEE Cloud Computing, 5*(1), 31–37.

Hardin, T., & Kotz, D. (2019). Blockchain in health data systems: A survey. *2019 Sixth International Conference on Internet of Things: Systems, Management and Security (IOTSMS)*, Granada, Spain, pp. 490–497.

Hasselgren, A., Kralevska, K., Gligoroski, D., Pedersen, S.A., & Faxvaag, A. (2020). Blockchain in healthcare and health sciences: A scoping review. *International Journal of Medical Informatics, 134*, 104040.

Idrees, S.M., Nowostawski, M., & Jameel, R. (2021). Blockchain-based digital contact tracing apps for COVID-19 pandemic management: Issues, challenges, solutions, and future directions. *JMIR Medical Informatics*, *9*(2), e25245.

Ismail, L., Materwala, H., & Zeadally, S. (2019). Lightweight blockchain for healthcare. *IEEE Access*, *7*, 149935–149951.

Khezr, S., Moniruzzaman, M., Yassine, A., & Benlamri, R. (2019). Blockchain technology in healthcare: A comprehensive review and directions for future research. *Applied Sciences*, *9*(9), 1736.

Qiu, J., Liang, X., Shetty, S., & Bowden, D. (2018). Towards secure and smart healthcare in smart cities using blockchain. *2018 IEEE International Smart Cities Conference (ISC2)*, Kansas City, Missouri, 1–4.

Ramani, V., Kumar, T., Bracken, A., Liyanage, M., & Ylianttila, M. (2018). Secure and efficient data accessibility in blockchain based healthcare systems. *2018 IEEE Global Communications Conference (GLOBECOM)*, Abu Dhabi, pp. 206–212.

Saha, A., Amin, R., Kunal, S., Vollala, S., & Dwivedi, S.K. (2019). Review on "Blockchain technology based medical healthcare system with privacy issues." *Security and Privacy*, *2*(5), e83.

Swathi, S., Sujithra, K., Sowmya, R., & Madhumathi, C.S. (2019). Secure health care data using blockchain: A survey. *International Research Journal of Engineering and Technology (IRJET)*, *6*(1), 1667–1671.

Zaghloul, E., Li, T., & Ren, J. (2019). Security and privacy of electronic health records: Decentralized and hierarchical data sharing using smart contracts. *2019 International Conference on Computing, Networking and Communications (ICNC)*, Honolulu, Hawaii, pp. 375–379.

12 Security and Privacy Concerns for Blockchain While Handling Healthcare Data

Rameez Yousuf and Dawood Ashraf Khan
University of Kashmir

Zubair Jeelani
Islamic University of Science and Technology

CONTENTS

12.1 INTRODUCTION

Healthcare systems are data-intensive systems in which medical data are generated, accessed, and disseminated in high frequencies. Digitization of the healthcare system is an obvious outcome of the development of health information systems that cater specific requirements of a healthcare facility. Initiatives have been taken by many countries and their governments to digitize the health data of patients in standard formats like electronic health records (EHRs), electronic medical records (EMRs), and personal health records (PHRs) to achieve specific objectives. For example, EMRs are more focused on extracting patient data for medical examination whereas PHR applications are used by patients to record their own medical data with the option of sharing this data with healthcare providers.

DOI: 10.1201/9781003141471-12

EHR system management solutions that rely on the traditional client–server or cloud suffer from issues of single point of failure, system vulnerability, data privacy, and centralized data stewardship [1]. Blockchain is a trustworthy distributed ledger database, consisting of a sequence of blocks that can be used to design an effective distributed system for healthcare that can withstand single point of failure effectively. The rest of this chapter is organized as follows: We begin with the introduction of EHR and EHR systems in Section 12.2; Section 12.3 discusses blockchain technology with emphasis on its application in healthcare; Section 12.4 presents the review of different state-of-the-art blockchain-based healthcare systems with a focus on security and privacy of sensitive health data; Section 12.5 discusses different research opportunities and practical challenges of blockchain technology adoption in healthcare; finally, the work is summarized in Section 12.6.

12.2 ELECTRONIC HEALTH RECORD SYSTEMS

EHRs are longitudinal patient health records that consist of a comprehensive clinical summary of the patient generated by one or more contacts with a healthcare facility. EHRs carry information pertaining to patient demographics, problems, past medical history, medications, vital signs, immunizations, laboratory data, and radiology reports [2]. EHR systems provide a patient's previous medical record history and ensure medical data consistency by avoiding redundancy as there is only one modifiable medical data file. EHRs can be shared among different healthcare facilities in a collaborative fashion to discover useful patterns from the data and discover useful knowledge that can be used for medical diagnosis and research. However, there are serious security and privacy challenges while sharing sensitive medical data among untrusted or semitrusted parties.

Different policies and laws have been adopted by different countries for maintaining the security and privacy of data. Data security and privacy policies and laws adopted by various countries are given in Table 12.1. Many reports in the last few years suggest some serious security and privacy breaches in the health data of patients. According to a report by the Centers for Medicare and Medicaid Services, the medical record of around 75,000 individuals was compromised in October 2018 [6]. According to another report published by Social Indicators Research, the record of over 173 million individuals was breached from October 2008 to September 2017 [7].

12.3 BLOCKCHAIN

Blockchain is a digital architecture in which transactions are recorded in the form of blocks that are linked together to create a digital chain of a distributed ledger as shown in Figure 12.1. All copies of the ledger are in sync and consensus all the time, eliminating the need for reconciliation and delays in processing in a distributed environment. Blockchain contains a number of blocks that are linked together in chronological order to create a chain that is practically immutable and is append-only. The first block in the blockchain is called "the genesis block" and does not contain any

TABLE 12.1

Data Privacy Laws in Various Countries

Country	Law	Highlights
USA	The Health Insurance Portability and Accountability Act (HIPAA) The Patient Safety and Quality Improvement Act of 2005 (PSQIA) Health Information Technology for Economic and Clinical Health (HITECH) Act of 2009	HIPAA passed in 1996 guarantees healthcare privacy in the United States. HIPAA can be divided into two components: HIPAA security rule—focuses on securing the electronic health information; and HIPAA privacy rule—focuses on protecting the privacy of health information like medical records, insurance information, and other patient specific details. The main objective of PSQIA is to improve patient safety by encouraging confidential reporting of events that adversely affect patients. Patient safety organizations are developed to gather, aggregate, and analyze the private and confidential information reported by healthcare facilities. HITECH Act further increases the scope of security and privacy protections available under HIPAA. HITECH provides increased legal liabilities for noncompliance and more stringent enforcement.
Canada	The Personal Information Protection and Electronic Documents Act (PIPEDA)	PIPEDA gives individuals the right to know the reasons for collection or use of their personal information. PIPEDA as such enforces organizations to enforce protection of this information in a secure manner. [3]
Brazil	The Brazilian Constitution, Article 5, Paragraph X Law 13.709 of Brazil (*Lei Geral de Proteção de Dados Pessoais* ("LGPD"))	The Brazilian Constitution ensures the inviolability of privacy, intimacy, and honor as a fundamental right. [4] LGPD is the general law for the protection of personal data sanctioned in August 2018. LGPD provides data subjects with nine rights, defines what constitutes personal data, and creates ten legal bases for lawful processing of personal data. Article 3 of LGPD outlines that the law applies to data processing pertaining to individuals within the territory of Brazil irrespective of if the data processing is done within or outside Brazil.
EU	Data Protection Directive (Directive 95/45/EC) The General Data Protection Regulation (GDPR)	Data Protection Directive is concerned with regulating personal data processing within the European Union and free data movement. GDPR was adopted in 2016 and it superseded the Data Protection Directive that was enforced in May 2018. Major highlights of GDPR include educating the users about data collection and handling processes; notifying users about the reasons for handling their data; getting prior consent to handle users' data; anonymizing gathered records; allowing users to withdraw their consent to data processing; notifying users of any breaches; giving users access to records; ensuring safe data transfers across borders and deleting information upon request.

(Continued)

TABLE 12.1 (*Continued*)
Data Privacy Laws in Various Countries

Country	Law	Highlights
UK	Data Protection Act 2018 (DPA)	DPA is the UK's implementation of GDPR. DPA regulates the use of personal information used by different organizations as well as the government. Entities using personal data have to follow "data protection principles" and must ensure that the information is used fairly, transparently, and lawfully; the purpose of information usage is specified explicitly and the information is used to a limit that is adequate, relevant, and limited to only what is necessary and is kept for no longer than is required. The information must be handled to ensure security.
Russia	Russian Federal Law on Personal Data (No. 152-FZ)	Implemented on July 27, 2006, the law contains the following highlights. Consent of individuals is necessary before their personal data can be processed. The individual must be informed about the operator and the prospective processing of the personal data. In case the data of an individual is migrated outside Russia, the operator must make sure that the rights of personal data subjects are sufficiently and adequately protected in the destination country.
India	Information Technology Act, 2000 (ITA-2000 or IT Act)	ITA-2000 is the primary law concerning electronic commerce and cybercrime in India. The major amendment to ITA-2000 was made in 2008.
	IT (Amendment) Act 2008	Handling of sensitive personal data or information by body corporates (companies like firm or sole proprietor) and liabilities to pay damages by way of compensation in case there is a wrongful loss or wrongful gain to any person.
China	Cyber Security Law (China Internet Security Law)	Focuses on protection and localization of data and cybersecurity in the interest of national security. [5]

previous hash as shown in Figure 12.1. Block 1 contains its data, hash, and hash of the previous block (genesis block). Block 2 contains its data, hash, and hash of block 1 and similarly block n contains its data, hash, and hash of block $n - 1$.

Blockchain technology is best suited in an untrustworthy peer-to-peer network without the need for a centralized authority. The trust in such an environment is determined by means of consensus algorithms which allow reaching an agreement on a certain value/state among the nodes in a network. The consensus algorithms in a blockchain network validate and verify the transactions, establish trust, and achieve reliability in such a decentralized network. Quite a good number of consensus algorithms have been proposed in the literature viz. Proof of Work [8], Proof of Stake [9], Delegated Proof-of-Stake [10], Proof of Authority [11], Proof of Burn [12], Proof of Identity [13], and Proof of Time [14].

Blockchain technology is beyond cryptocurrencies and finds multiuse cases in healthcare sector [15–17], insurance [18,19], finance [20,21], supply chain [22,23,53],

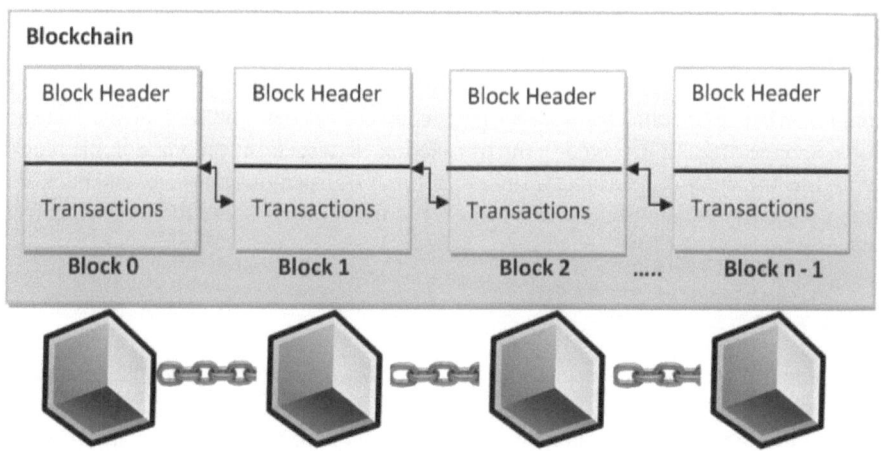

FIGURE 12.1   Blockchain architecture.

entertainment [24,25], gaming [26,27], internet of things (IoT) [28,29], voting [30,31], agriculture, [32,33] and crowd funding [34].

12.3.1   FEATURES OF BLOCKCHAIN

Blockchain technology is characterized by certain features like decentralized, immutable, secured, transparent, anonymous, and auditable [35].

Decentralized: Blockchain is decentralized in nature where there is no central authority that governs the operations in the network which consists of peer-to-peer nodes. The transactions between these nodes do not require any central authority (e.g., a bank) to validate them; rather the transactions are validated among the nodes in the network. As a result of this mode of operation in the blockchain network, the issues of performance bottleneck and single point of failure are handled effectively.

Immutable: Once the records are added in a block, they cannot be altered or modified. The records in a blockchain are immutable and are append-only.

Secured: Blockchain is secured by design as the records in a block cannot be tampered with. It is practically impossible to tamper with any block in a blockchain as the blocks are linked together with cryptographic hash functions. If a block is altered, it will change the hash of that block and the following blocks will become invalid. The attacker will need to change the hash of all the following blocks which is practically impossible as it will require huge computational power and a lot of computations.

Transparent: The best part of blockchain technology lies in its ability to be transparent. The transactions/records in a blockchain are visible to any individual who has downloaded the blockchain on his/her computer system.

Anonymous: A blockchain user is given a public/private key pair with which the user can transact in a blockchain network. When a user wants to make a transaction, the user uses this key pair in the form of hashes to transact between parties in which the user addresses are hashed. It becomes difficult for the users in the blockchain network to identify who is transacting to whom, thus providing a good level of anonymity to the users.

Auditable*:* The transactions in a blockchain are time-stamped, providing information when a specific transaction has occurred, parties involved in the transaction, and the amount involved in the transaction. Transactions recorded in the blocks with this information facilitate a smooth audit of transactions on the blockchain. For example, party A cannot deny that party B has not sent (say some Bitcoins) if, in fact, party B has sent the Bitcoins to party A.

12.3.2 CLASSIFICATION OF BLOCKCHAIN

Blockchain systems can be classified into public, private, or consortium based on user access.

Public Blockchain*:* A public blockchain is an open, permissionless network that allows anyone to join the network and to have access to the blockchain contents. It is truly a decentralized network that is not governed by a single entity. Examples: Bitcoin and Ethereum [36].

Private Blockchain*:* A private blockchain is a permissioned network that restricts the addition of users to the network; only authorized users have access to the network. It is a bit of a more centralized network that is controlled by one or more entities. Examples: Ripple [37] and Hyperledger [38].

Consortium Blockchain: A consortium blockchain is a permissioned network in which there are multiple entities that govern the network. It is partially decentralized in the sense that only a selected set of nodes participates in the consensus determination. Examples: Quorum [39] and Corda [37].

12.3.3 SMART CONTRACT

Smart contracts are self-executing pieces of code that get executed automatically when a predefined condition is met at a given time and updates the blockchain instantly. The use of smart contracts streamlines the process (e.g., buying and selling of a car), eliminates the need for a third party to execute the terms listed in an agreement, and saves time and money. Smart contracts find applications in mortgage payment, insurance, and e-commerce [40]. Some smart contract platforms are Ethereum, EOS, Stellar [41], NEO [42], and Hyperledger Fabric [43].

12.3.4 DIGITAL SIGNATURE

A digital signature uses asymmetric cryptography to authenticate transactions in a blockchain network. The transaction is first signed by the sender's private key, then the transaction is broadcasted over the blockchain network, and finally, the public key of the sender is used by all other nodes in the network to verify the authenticity of the received transaction. Once the verification process is successful, the transaction is added to the blockchain network. Presently, the blockchain network uses elliptic curve digital signature algorithm [44].

12.3.5 Blockchain in Healthcare

EHR is digital information of a patient's medical history stored centrally, which can be retrieved while treating a patient and prescribing the medicine or can be used for research purposes also. Health information exchange (HIE) is the movement of EHR records among hospitals or organizations. The problem with HIE that may arise is information blockage that happens when a hospital does not want to share patients' records with other hospitals; another problem is data corruption, as anyone can have access to the data and can tamper the data easily. There are also high chances of privacy breach as patients' EHR can be compromised for some gains by interested parties. Blockchain technology comes as a savior to address the issues of security and privacy in healthcare data.

12.4 STATE-OF-THE-ART BLOCKCHAIN-BASED EHR SYSTEMS

One of the most important applications of blockchain technology is in the field of healthcare. EHRs are used to examine a variety of medical conditions in patients. The security and privacy of such medical data are of utmost importance. Recently, various blockchain-based solutions have been proposed to maintain the security and privacy of healthcare data. This section presents a review of state-of-the-art blockchain-based healthcare systems with an emphasis on the security and privacy of healthcare data. A quick summary of these techniques is presented in Table 12.2.

The work presented in Ref. [45] proposes a model to use blockchain and cloud storage to guarantee that the security and privacy of patients' records remain intact while sharing EHR among medical institutions. The EHR ciphertext which is provided by data providers (e.g., hospital) is stored in the cloud server and the EHR indexes are stored on the blockchain. The data security is provided by means of keyword searchable encryption, while privacy preservation is guaranteed by employing proxy re-encryption. The data owners remain in control of their data, and the data could be shared among hospitals only after getting consent from the data owner. The data requestor needs to first get the search trapdoor from the data provider and then searches for keywords in the blockchain. Then, the data requester sends a request for EHR to the data owner; if the data owner accepts the request to share its EHR, only then the data requester will get the re-encrypted EHR from the cloud server.

Authors in Ref. [46] propose a blockchain framework in collaboration with interplanetary file system (IPFS) for the storage and retrieval of EHRs. The IPFS protocol is used for secure data storage and data sharing in a blockchain environment. The IPFS protocol uses "content-based addressing" rather than "location-based addressing" and stores the hash of files stored on it. This protocol stores only a single copy of a file, thus ensuring storage efficiency. In the proposed model, EHRs are stored in IPFS in the form of hashes; the role-based access control mechanisms are used to define who can view the data, thus ensuring that the unauthorized users do not have access to the EHR of patients. Only the doctors and patients have access to the data, thereby ensuring the security and privacy of data.

TABLE 12.2
Summary of the Blockchain-Based Healthcare Systems

Work	Technologies Implemented	Storage	Security	Privacy	Blockchain Platform
Wang et al. [45]	Consortium blockchain	Cloud	Searchable encryption and conditional proxy re-encryption	Searchable encryption and conditional proxy re-encryption	Ethereum
Shahnaz et al. [46]	Blockchain	IPFS	Role-based access control	Smart contracts	Ethereum
Esposito et al. [47]	Blockchain	Cloud	Consensus algorithms	Blockchain	-
Tanwar et al. [48]	Blockchain	Blockchain	Access control policies	Access control policies	Hyperledger Fabric and Hyperledger Composer
Ismail et al. [49]	Permissioned blockchain	Blockchain	Practical byzantine fault tolerance permissioned blockchain	Permissioned blockchain, canals	Architecture simulated on NS3 simulator
Pandey and Litoriya [50]	Permissioned blockchain	Blockchain	Public key cryptography permissioned blockchain	Pseudonymity (hash of patient ID is used to identify the patient record) contract confidentiality	Hyperledger fabric
Omar et al. [51]	Blockchain	Blockchain, cloud	User authentication encryption	Pseudonymity (dynamic keys)	-
Fu et al. [52]	Blockchain	Blockchain	EMR shares	Interleaving encoding	-

In Ref. [47], the authors discuss the issues with the cloud being centralized in nature; the data stored therein is vulnerable to attacks (both inside and outside), performance bottleneck, and single point of failure. Blockchain technology is used for storing the EHRs in a decentralized manner and addresses the issues with centralized cloud storage. Blockchain gives patients control over their own data and keeps the data stored in an immutable format, as a result of which the security and privacy of patients' EHR is maintained. The work further discusses the challenges with the blockchain technology such as storage issues and proposes to use off-chain storage with the blockchain.

The work presented in Ref. [48] proposes a framework for the healthcare system using blockchain technology where participants like patients, clinicians, lab, and system admin need to register for an enrollment certificate using membership service provider from the certificate authority. The participant is given a certificate and a private key with a new ID and enrolls participants. Some smart contracts defined in the proposed framework are CreateMedicalRecord, GrantAccessToClinician, GrantAccessToLab, RevokeAccess, and RevokeAccessToLab. Different roles for the participants have been defined which limits their access to the records in the Hyperledger Fabric blockchain. When a patient adds a record by means of a client application, the chain code for Hyperledger Fabric is invoked for a transaction to be committed in the blockchain network. Once the transaction is committed, it is distributed over the whole network and every participant gets an updated record of the patient. This approach ensures that an unauthorized user cannot have access to records to update or delete any of these.

A patient is given a private key and the patient has to read, write, and revoke EHR accesses in the proposed framework. A patient's record M_{PID} can be accessed by the clinicians or labs only if the patient grants access to these participants. These participants can then view or update the patient's record in the blockchain network. The proposed framework has access control policies by which it ensures the security and privacy of the patients' EHRs.

Work presented in Ref. [49] discusses a lightweight blockchain-based healthcare data management system with a focus on reducing the communication as well as the computational overhead when compared to Bitcoin-based blockchain networks. The whole network is divided into clusters, and each cluster maintains a copy of the ledger. The use of a permissioned blockchain network is used to get around the problems that can occur if permissionless blockchain network is used like unauthorized network participation, impersonation, privacy issues, and slow throughput. Different components of the proposed architecture include head blockchain manager (HBCM), blockchain manager (BCM), canal, ledger (L), notification manager (NM), and consensus.

HBCM in the proposed architecture is responsible for the overall management of the blockchain network. HBCM has the following responsibilities: HBCM provides a valid digital identity to the participants on the network and the transactions carried out by different clients are received by HBCM and generate blocks. The use of a single HBCM for mining reduces the computational effort and energy consumption otherwise present in Bitcoin networks. Clients on the proposed network submit transactions to the HBCM that enters the transactions into a ledger (L). In order to enhance the reliability of the system and to avoid single point of failure, two HBCMs, namely leader and follower, are used. The leader is responsible for block generation and the follower receives the blocks from the leader and replicates them. There is no need for forking in the architecture because all the blocks are generated by the HBCM, therefore minimizing both effort and time.

The architecture divides the hospitals (participants) into clusters based on their demography and a node in the network is designated as the cluster node. The ledger is maintained by the cluster node, therefore minimizing the data communication overhead that would be otherwise needed to communicate with each node in the network. The designated cluster node is referred to as BCM that takes part in consensus and maintains a copy of the ledger on the network. A ledger of valid transactions and invalid transactions is maintained by the BCM by verifying the blocks received from HBCM. The architecture uses a permissioned network to enhance the security and privacy of sensitive medical data. The concept of a canal is used to facilitate communication between a subset of nodes in the permissioned network to perform some confidential transactions. Copies of ledger are maintained by HBCMs and BCMs. The invalid transactions are recorded in the ledger for auditing purposes. NM within a BCM is responsible for handling the notification of different events in the network. The architecture uses the practical Byzantine fault tolerance (PBFT) consensus protocol. Consistent prefix and monotonic prefix consistency (MPC) is used as replication strategies in this architecture.

The proposed architecture is compared with the Bitcoin blockchain network. Experimental results reveal 11 times less network traffic with the proposed architecture when compared with the Bitcoin network and 1.13 times faster ledger updates. The proposed blockchain network has low computational and communication overhead as compared to the Bitcoin network. The PBFT consensus protocol used is scalable and energy-efficient. Division of network into clusters and maintenance of BCMs considerably reduces communication delay and computational effort, making the architecture more scalable. The issues of forking are addressed by delegating the generation of blocks to HBCMs. The use of permissioned network and robust replication strategies ensure data privacy and security.

Work proposed in Ref. [50] discusses a blockchain-based architecture that is sufficiently modified to meet the specific requirements of e-healthcare systems. The proposed architecture uses the Hyperledger Fabric by IBM because of its computational efficiency and confidentiality and also because it keeps the contract confidential between the two parties involved in the contract. The architecture being distributed is robust against single point of failure. Participating nodes maintain a ledger of all transactions in the network. The architecture identifies five types of nodes: clients, representatives, coordinators, organizers, and committers.

Client nodes place their requests on the network for required services. The representative nodes are responsible for handling and validating client requests. Coordinator nodes verify the client's request endorsements and reject or accept proposals for further ordering. Organizer nodes get the verified proposals from the coordinator nodes and generate blocks to organize transactions within the blocks. Organizer nodes also broadcast the newly generated blocks in the network. Authentication and Authority Agency (AAA) provides identification for each entity on the network. As such, only AAA verified entities are allowed to perform different tasks as per the authorized access given to each entity.

The proposed architecture sets a size of 20 KB for the blocks and also places a time limit of 5 minutes after which the blocks are committed in the ledger. Therefore, the problem of undermined time to commit the blocks is addressed. The security of the network is maintained by allowing only authorized parties to propose or look into different transactions. The privacy of the patient is ensured by removing the identifying information from patient data. Patient ID provided by AAA is hashed and this hash is used to identify documents pertaining to a specific patient. The proposed architecture is designed to incorporate some important features that make it scalable, robust, business-oriented, transparent, and private. Public key cryptography can be used to facilitate HIE, transaction verification, and nonrepudiation by the sender.

Work presented in Ref. [51] proposes a platform for the storage of healthcare data to retain data privacy using a blockchain-based environment. The proposed platform is shown to maintain the security and privacy of data by utilizing the blockchain technology and cryptographic functions to ensure pseudonymity. The protocol proposed in this work is called MediBChain protocol. The proposed platform recognizes different entities and roles as follows. Patients assume the role of a data sender that sends their personal healthcare data to the system in an encrypted form. The data receivers request data and are granted access to the requested data only after they are successfully authenticated. Authentication of data senders and data receivers is the responsibility of the registration unit. Users in the system are authenticated using a user ID and a password provided by the registration unit. The private accessible unit facilitates secure interaction between the elements at different levels in the system. Blockchain is meant to store user data in the system. Each transaction in the blockchain returns a transaction identifier. Transaction identifier is used to access further data by the user. The system uses a permissioned blockchain that requires authentication for data access.

Pseudonymity is provided by the system to hide the identity of the data sender and the data receiver from all parties in the system during a transaction. The data sent to the system by a data sender is encrypted and identification-less attributes in the data help achieve pseudonymity. The data receiver uses a block hash to trace a particular block in the blockchain that holds the private data of the data sender. The privacy of the system is maintained because the hash of each block is unique and is associated with unique parties in the system. Only data stored in the block are accessible to the specific party.

Authors in Ref. [52] propose use of blockchain technology in combination with a lightweight message sharing to share a patient's EMR while preserving data integrity, security, and patient's privacy. In the proposed framework, the creation of EMR shares, their storage, recovery, and usage of EMRs are defined. In the first phase, i.e., creation and storage of EMR shares, the shares are stored in the blockchain rather than the plaintext EMR. The original plaintext EMR of length l is divided into l/t groups, with each group containing t bits. By means of interleaving encoding, we get t sub-messages $(x_1, x_2, ..., x_t)$ which are semantically not meaningful even if the malicious actor gets these sub-messages.

The n EMR shares s_i $(i = 1, 2, ..., n)$ are constructed from t sub-messages in the encrypted form which further enhances the privacy of users. The encrypted EMR shares are forwarded to the nodes in the blockchain environment where these are stored. The healthcare blockchain system stores the indexes of these EMR shares. The EMR shares and their identifiers are broadcasted to the whole blockchain network for verification. After the verification process, the EMR shares are stored in the form of blocks in the blockchain network.

When a user requests for EMR of a patient, the user has to first search for the index of the EMR on the blockchain and search at least t nodes in the blockchain network that stores the shares of the EMR. The user collects a subset of EMR shares and then reconstructs the original EMR by applying a coefficient matrix. The result of this process is the creation of subsections $(x_1, x_2, ..., x_t)$. This process improves the efficiency of the verification and recovery process of EMR reconstruction. The recovery process is followed by decoding of the EMR subsections obtained from the reconstruction process. The interleaving decoder translates the EMR subsections into the original EMR which can later be used by doctors, patients, and insurance agencies or for research purposes.

The proposed method preserves the security and privacy of a patient's medical data because an attacker cannot reveal the original EMR after getting the EMR shares from the blockchain nodes as it does not have the knowledge of interleaving encoding rules. Moreover, an attacker cannot tamper with the EMRs as the mining nodes will not allow modification of the EMRs.

EHR systems hosted on a centralized cloud server suffer from issues like single point of failure and security and privacy of sensitive patient data. Blockchain technology has been employed to implement EHR systems that ensure the security and privacy of healthcare data. However, there are some issues inherent to the blockchain technology like limited storage capacity, lack of user authentication in case of permissionless blockchain and lack of role-based authentication of users in case of permissioned blockchain. The issue of limited storage has been addressed by proposing IPFS or cloud storage systems to save patient data off-chain and store only indexes of records in the blockchain. Authentication of users is mostly done using permissioned blockchain, role-based, and certificate-based user authentication. Cryptographic functions are also used in many techniques to ensure the pseudonymity of patients in the blockchain network. The use of smart contracts to commit health-related transactions in the system facilitates verification of these transactions to ensure security, privacy, and consistency of the data. Review of state-of-the-art techniques presented in this section shows the potential of using blockchain technology in healthcare and the resolution of most of the issues prevalent in the current healthcare solutions.

12.5   RESEARCH OPPORTUNITIES AND PRACTICAL CHALLENGES

Academic research has focused on employing blockchain technology in healthcare to solve specific problems like security and privacy. The solutions seem promising to be used in a practical setup, but there are certain research opportunities and challenges that must be addressed to witness a shift from traditional EHR systems to blockchain-based EHR systems. Blockchain technology is fundamentally computationally expensive and requiring large bandwidth. Researchers are working in this area and trying to tailor the blockchain to meet the requirements of healthcare industries to reduce the computation and bandwidth requirements to allow the scalability of these systems. Integration of machine learning with blockchain-based systems can result in wonderful outcomes if the health data stored with blockchain can be presented to machine learning models in a proper format. Efforts have been made in this direction, and many researchers have made attempts to integrate machine learning with blockchain technology to extract invaluable information from the health data available. The issues of limited storage on blockchain have been worked out by the researchers, and the use of IPFS, cloud, and off-chain databases has been proposed as a solution. Quick adoption of IoT in healthcare and large-scale use of things like sensors pose serious security threats to patient privacy. Blockchain-based solutions can be explored to better manage these things so that security of these devices is ensured.

12.6 SUMMARY

This chapter presents a review of different EHR management systems based on blockchain technology. Problems with centralized EHR management are highlighted and the motivation behind using blockchain technology for the purpose is discussed. Different state-of-the-art blockchain-based EHR systems proposed recently are discussed with emphasis on the mechanisms to achieve health data security and privacy in these systems. Finally, the research opportunities and practical challenges for using blockchain technology in healthcare are discussed.

REFERENCES

1. Ismail, L., Materwala, H., & Zeadally, S. (2019). Lightweight blockchain for healthcare. *IEEE Access*, 7, 149935–149951. doi:10.1109/access.2019.2947613.
2. Menachemi, N., & Collum. (2011). Benefits and drawbacks of electronic health record systems. *Risk Management and Healthcare Policy*, 4, 47. doi:10.2147/rmhp.s12985.
3. Jensen, M. (2013). Challenges of privacy protection in big data analytics. *2013 IEEE International Congress on Big Data*. doi:10.1109/bigdata.congress.2013.39.
4. Fortes, V. B., Oro Boff, S., & Galindo Ayuda, F. (2016). The fundamental right to privacy in Brazil and the internet privacy rights in regulating personal data protection. *Revista Eletrônica Do Curso de Direito Da UFSM*, 11(1), 24. doi:10.5902/1981369419706.
5. Wagner, J. "China's cybersecurity law: What you need to know." The Diplomat. June 01, 2017. Accessed November 20, 2020. https://thediplomat.com/2017/06/chinas-cybersecurity-law-what-you-need-to-know/.
6. Caffery, M. "CMS reports data breach in ACA and broker portal." www.ajmc.com. October 23, 2018. Accessed October 22, 2020. https://www.ajmc.com/view/cms-reports-data-breach-in-aca-breach-in-aca-agent-and-broker-portal.
7. Koczkodaj, W. W., Mazurek, M., Strzałka, D., Wolny-Dominiak, A., & Woodbury-Smith, M. (2018). Electronic health record breaches as social indicators. *Social Indicators Research*, 141(2), 861–871. doi:10.1007/s11205-018-1837-z.
8. van Tilborg, H. C. A., Sushil Jajodia (Eds.) (2011). Proof of work. In *Encyclopedia of Cryptography and Security*, pp. 984–984. Springer, Boston, MA. doi: 10.1007/978-1-4419-5906-5_1060.
9. Saleh, F. (2018). Blockchain without waste: Proof-of-stake. *SSRN Electronic Journal*. doi: 10.2139/ssrn.3183935.
10. Tan, C., & Xiong, L. (2020, June). DPoSB: Delegated proof of stake with node's behavior and Borda Count. *In 2020 IEEE 5th Information Technology and Mechatronics Engineering Conference (ITOEC)*, Chongqing, China (pp. 1429–1434), IEEE.
11. Tempesta, S. (2019). Deploy ethereum proof-of-authority. *Introduction to Blockchain for Azure Developers*. doi:10.1007/978-1-4842-5311-3_2.
12. Karantias, K., Kiayias, A., & Zindros, D. (2020). Proof-of-burn. *Lecture Notes in Computer Science*, 523–540. doi:10.1007/978-3-030-51280-4_28.

13. Cerezo Sánchez, D. (2019). Zero-knowledge proof-of-identity: Sybil-resistant, anonymous authentication on permissionless blockchains and incentive compatible, strictly dominant cryptocurrencies. *SSRN Electronic Journal.* doi:10.2139/ssrn.3392331.

14. Chen, L., Xu, L., Shah, N., Gao, Z., Lu, Y., & Shi, W. (2017, November). On security analysis of proof-of-elapsed-time (poet). *In International Symposium on Stabilization, Safety, and Security of Distributed Systems,* Springer, Cham, (pp. 282–297).

15. Abdellatif, A. A., Al-Marridi, A. Z., Mohamed, A., Erbad, A., Chiasserini, C. F., & Refaey, A. (2020). ssHealth: Toward secure, blockchain-enabled healthcare systems. *IEEE Network,* 34(4), 312–319. doi:10.1109/mnet.011.1900553.

16. Idrees, S. M., Nowostawski, M., & Jameel, R. (2021). Blockchain-based digital contact tracing apps for COVID-19 pandemic management: Issues, challenges, solutions, and future directions. *JMIR Medical Informatics,* 9(2), e25245.

17. Idrees, S.M., Nowostawski, M., Jameel, R., Mourya, A.K. 2021. 7 privacy-preserving. In *Data Protection and Privacy in Healthcare: Research and Innovations,* CRC Press, Boca Raton, FL, p. 109.

18. Sun, J., Yao, X., Wang, S., & Wu, Y. (2020). Non-repudiation storage and access control scheme of insurance data based on blockchain in IPFS. *IEEE Access,* 8, 155145–155155. doi:10.1109/access.2020.3018816.

19. Raikwar, M., Mazumdar, S., Ruj, S., Gupta, S. S., Chattopadhyay, A., & Lam, K. Y. (2018, February). A blockchain framework for insurance processes. *In 2018 9th IFIP International Conference on New Technologies, Mobility and Security (NTMS),* IEEE, pp. 1–4.

20. Ahluwalia, S., Mahto, R. V., & Guerrero, M. (2020). Blockchain technology and startup financing: A transaction cost economics perspective. *Technological Forecasting and Social Change,* 151, 119854. doi:10.1016/j.techfore.2019.119854.

21. Treleaven, P., Brown, R. G., & Yang, D. (2017). Blockchain technology in finance. *Computer,* 50(9), 14–17.

22. Liu, Z., & Li, Z. (2020). A blockchain-based framework of cross-border e-commerce supply chain. *International Journal of Information Management,* 52, 102059. doi:10.1016/j.ijinfomgt.2019.102059.

23. Saberi, S., Kouhizadeh, M., Sarkis, J., & Shen, L. (2019). Blockchain technology and its relationships to sustainable supply chain management. *International Journal of Production Research,* 57(7), 2117–2135.

24. Liao, D.-Y., & Wang, X. (2018). Applications of blockchain technology to logistics management in integrated casinos and entertainment. *Informatics,* 5(4), 44. doi:10.3390/informatics5040044.

25. Tripathi, S. (2018, October). Blockchain application in media and entertainment. In *SMPTE* 2018 (pp. 1–8), Los Angeles, CA. doi: 10.5594/M001857

26. Wu, F., Yuen, H. Y., Chan, H. C. B., Leung, V. C. M., & Cai, W. (2020). Infinity battle: A glance at how blockchain techniques serve in a serverless gaming system. *Proceedings of the 28th ACM International Conference on Multimedia.* doi:10.1145/3394171.3414458.

27. Yuen, H. Y., Wu, F., Cai, W., Chan, H. C., Yan, Q., & Leung, V. C. (2019, July). Proof-of-play: A novel consensus model for blockchain-based peer-to-peer gaming system. *In Proceedings of the 2019 ACM International Symposium on Blockchain and Secure Critical Infrastructure* (pp. 19–28).

28. Banafa, A. (2017). IoT and blockchain convergence: Benefits and challenges. IEEE Internet of Things.

29. Samaniego, M., Jamsrandorj, U., & Deters, R. (2016, December). Blockchain as a service for IoT. *In 2016 IEEE International Conference on Internet of Things (iThings) and IEEE Green Computing and Communications (GreenCom) and IEEE Cyber, Physical and Social Computing (CPSCom) and IEEE Smart Data (SmartData),* (pp. 433–436), Chengdu, China, IEEE.

30. Khan, K. M., Arshad, J., & Khan, M. M. (2020). Investigating performance constraints for blockchain based secure e-voting system. *Future Generation Computer Systems*, 105, 13–26. doi:10.1016/j.future.2019.11.005.
31. Kshetri, N., & Voas, J. (2018). Blockchain-enabled e-voting. *IEEE Software*, 35(4), 95–99.
32. Kamilaris, A., Fonts, A., & Prenafeta-Boldú, F. X. (2019). The rise of blockchain technology in agriculture and food supply chains. *Trends in Food Science & Technology*, 91, 640–652.
33. Papa, S. F. (2017, June). Use of blockchain technology in agribusiness: Transparency and monitoring in agricultural trade. *In 2017 International Conference on Management Science and Management Innovation (MSMI 2017)*, Suzhou, China, Atlantis Press.
34. Miraz, M. H., & Ali, M. (2018). Applications of blockchain technology beyond cryptocurrency. *Annals of Emerging Technologies in Computing*, 2(1), 1–6. doi:10.33166/aetic.2018.01.001.
35. Zheng, Z., Xie, S., Dai, H., Chen, X., & Wang, H. (2017). An overview of blockchain technology: Architecture, consensus, and future trends. *2017 IEEE International Congress on Big Data (BigData Congress)*. doi:10.1109/bigdatacongress.2017.85.
36. Gencer, A. E., Basu, S., Eyal, I., van Renesse, R., & Sirer, E. G. (2018). Decentralization in bitcoin and ethereum networks. *Lecture Notes in Computer Science*, 439–457. doi:10.1007/978-3-662-58387-6_24.
37. Benji, M., & Sindhu, M. (2018). A study on the Corda and ripple blockchain platforms. *Advances in Big Data and Cloud Computing*, 179–187. doi:10.1007/978-981-13-1882-5_16.
38. Krstić, M., & Krstić, L. (2020). Hyperledger frameworks with a special focus on hyperledger fabric. *Vojnotehnicki Glasnik*, 68(3), 639–663. doi:10.5937/vojtehg68-26206.
39. Baliga, A., Subhod, I., Kamat, P., & Chatterjee, S. (2018). Performance evaluation of the quorum blockchain platform. arXiv preprint arXiv:1809.03421.
40. Alharby, M., & van Moorsel, A. (2017). Blockchain based smart contracts: A systematic mapping study. *Computer Science & Information Technology (CS & IT)*. doi:10.5121/csit.2017.71011.
41. Barański, S., Szymański, J., Sobecki, A., Gil, D., & Mora, H. (2020). Practical I-voting on stellar blockchain. *Applied Sciences*, 10(21), 7606.
42. Coelho, I., Coelho, V., Lin, P., & Zhang, E. (2020). Community yellow paper: A technical specification for neo blockchain.
43. Aleksieva, V., Valchanov, H., & Huliyan, A. (2020). Implementation of smart-contract, based on hyperledger fabric blockchain. *2020 21st International Symposium on Electrical Apparatus & Technologies (SIELA)*. doi:10.1109/siela49118.2020.9167043.
44. Johnson, D., Menezes, A., & Vanstone, S. (2001). The Elliptic Curve Digital Signature Algorithm (ECDSA). *International Journal of Information Security*, 1(1), 36–63. doi:10.1007/s102070100002.
45. Wang, Y., Zhang, A., Zhang, P., & Wang, H. (2019). Cloud-assisted EHR sharing with security and privacy preservation via consortium blockchain. *IEEE Access*, 7, 136704–136719. doi:10.1109/access.2019.2943153.
46. Shahnaz, A., Qamar, U., & Khalid, A. (2019). Using blockchain for electronic health records. *IEEE Access*, 7, 147782–147795. doi:10.1109/access.2019.2946373.
47. Esposito, C., De Santis, A., Tortora, G., Chang, H., & Choo, K.-K. R. (2018). Blockchain: A panacea for healthcare cloud-based data security and privacy? *IEEE Cloud Computing*, 5(1), 31–37. doi:10.1109/mcc.2018.011791712.
48. Tanwar, S., Parekh, K., & Evans, R. (2020). Blockchain-based electronic healthcare record system for healthcare 4.0 applications. *Journal of Information Security and Applications*, 50, 102407. doi:10.1016/j.jisa.2019.102407.
49. Ismail, L., Materwala, H., & Zeadally, S. (2019). Lightweight blockchain for healthcare. *IEEE Access*, 7, 149935–149951. doi:10.1109/access.2019.2947613.

50. Pandey, P., & Litoriya, R. (2020). Securing and authenticating healthcare records through blockchain technology. *Cryptologia*, 44(4), 341–356. doi:10.1080/01611194.2019.1706060.

51. Omar, A. A., Bhuiyan, M. Z. A., Basu, A., Kiyomoto, S., & Rahman, M. S. (2019). Privacy-friendly platform for healthcare data in cloud based on blockchain environment. *Future Generation Computer Systems*, 95, 511–521. doi:10.1016/j.future.2018.12.044.

52. Fu, J., Wang, N., & Cai, Y. (2020). Privacy-preserving in healthcare blockchain systems based on lightweight message sharing. *Sensors*, 20(7), 1898. doi:10.3390/s20071898.

53. Idrees, S.M.; Nowostawski, M.; Jameel, R.; Mourya, A.K. Security Aspects of Blockchain Technology Intended for Industrial Applications. Electronics 2021, 10, 951. https://doi.org/10.3390/electronics10080951

13 Blockchain Technology in Medical Data Management and Protection in India
The Law in the Making

Shambhu Prasad Chakrabarty
and Souvik Mukherjee
The West Bengal National University of Juridical Sciences

CONTENTS

DOI: 10.1201/9781003141471-13

13.1   INTRODUCTION

In this study, we have researched medical data laws prevailing in India and try to analyse the position of blockchain technology in its domain. The paper is divided into five parts. The second part unravels briefly, the legal standing of healthcare data management and the use of technology in India, with the first introducing the paper. The third part explains the significant challenges that blockchain technology may face amidst the existing legal environment. The fourth part discusses the viability of blockchain technology and stratified various challenges in the traditional healthcare practice and system. The fifth part concludes the paper with a prelude to the beneficiaries of this strategic endeavour.

The methodology adopted in this paper incorporates drawing of conclusion using cross-country analysis for solutions to address the challenges brought forth by this complicated position.

The paper is based on primary and secondary sources in this genre of study.

The medical sector is undergoing a significant transformation induced by the rapid development of new technologies with blockchain technology being the recent entrant, after a considerable success of this technology in other sectors, including finance. This confusion of technology with the medical industry has already shown promising outcomes in some jurisdictions.

To start with, it is essential to unravel the mystery behind some terminology typically used in the domain of blockchain technology.

Smart Contracts: From a legal point of view, contracts are agreements enforceable by law. Prima facie, smart contracts seem to be a specie of the genus contract. However, on a closer look, it appears to be a misnomer. It is a part of the technology that would increase the efficiency in the healthcare industry. The technology would automate the requisite tasks and improve the efficacy of the system by removing the middlemen. This, consequently, would reduce the cost of the process. For instance, by applying this technology, the system automatically records the details of the care or treatment received by a patient [1,2]. Once connected, for example, with an insurance company, the intrinsic elements of each transaction do not require to be brought to the notice of the insurer as they can see it automatically, and once specific parameters are complied, a claim would be disbursed automatically.

Legally speaking, smart contracts are not agreements *per se* but are codes that implement the business logic involved in a standard contract. It has been seen that there is generally a contract in existence between the parties who invoke the smart contract between them. It is similar to auto bill pay, wherein the users enter into a "terms of service" leading to the generation of codes which implement the contract.

Another exciting term used in this domain is the distributed ledger technology (DLT). It refers to a new approach of recording and sharing data across data stores commonly known as ledgers. The process records, shares, and synchronises the data thus collected across the selected network participants.

TABLE 13.1

Legislations to Protect Data Privacy in India (Selected)

Sl. No.	Legislations (Selective)	Provisions (Selective)
1	Indian Telegraph Act, 1885 and Indian Telegraph Rules	Sections 4 and 5Rule 419A of the IT Rules
2	Indian Post Office Act, 1898	Section 26
3	The Indian Wireless Telegraphy Act, 1933	Sections 3 and 4 vesting the power on the Government to regulate data
4	Information Technology Act, 2000 and Information Technology Rules	Section 69
5	Unlawful Activities Prevention Act, 1967	Section 4
6	Code of Criminal Procedure, 1973	Section 91
7	Consumer Protection Act, 2019	Unfair Trade Practice to disclose the data of the consumers
8	Right to Information Act, 2005	Section 8 (including related provisions)
9	Personal Data Protection Bill, 2018	Yet to be enacted

13.2 POSITION OF HEALTHCARE DATA MANAGEMENT AND THE USE OF TECHNOLOGY IN INDIA

India is a new entrant when it comes to using technology in healthcare management. A brief study of the various models used in healthcare reveals the absence of any specific model which is full proof. However, it is clear that the conversion from purely mechanical models to electronic versions has been done. There is also an absence of any specific regulatory mechanism for collecting, storing or distributing medical data. However, Table 13.1 would act as a guideline relating to the existing laws pertaining to medical data privacy in India.

13.3 CHALLENGES OF USE OF TECHNOLOGY IN THE HEALTHCARE SECTOR

With the advent of technology, the healthcare sector has witnessed significant development. Globalisation and industrialisation have flooded the healthcare sector as they did to other areas of discourse. Blockchain technology in the healthcare industry is a new entrant. After the success of blockchain technology in finance (bitcoin), other sectors have discovered the potential to revolutionise through this technology as it would enable a lot of challenges involved in their system otherwise tough to manage.

Bereft of evolutionary potential, blockchain technology would have to fit in the existing legal setup, which is conservative in most jurisdictions. The significant issues in bringing this technology to the fore are the robust privacy rights regime with a centralised regulation on data protection law.

The United States of America and European region act as major players in this particular regime of blockchain, as they account for 9565 and 8265 projects respectively [18]. In the field of information technology, the General Data Protection Regulation, 2018 (GDPR) of European Union has contributed significantly the privacy concerns in the internet age by virtue of seven principles: lawfulness, fairness and transparency; purpose identification, limitation on data collection; accuracy; limitation and regulation on storage of data; integrity, confidentiality [2]; and accountability [4,5]. Even though the financial sector took lead in the development of blockchain and introduced bitcoins, a survey report of 200 healthcare executives spread across 16 countries conducted by the IBM Institute for Business Values stated that 16% of the survey has moved on from the experimentation with the technology in the healthcare sector and have commercial blockchain solution by 2017 (Health Europa, 2020). However, data security still remains one of the biggest roadblocks in the progress. In addition to the security issues which even if one could overcome, concerns remain regarding the scaling up of the technology. The regulation on data protection and privacy in Europe and United States, i.e. GDPR and HIPAA respectively [10,11], can come to aid substantially regarding the data protection concerns but that may not be enough looking at the volume of data [1,3]. Sui generis legislation addressing blockchain technology is desired but that awaits the substantial clarity in the application of the technology. Incidentally, European Parliament and European Commission brought forward a new regulation, nomenclature as Medical Devices Regulation, directed towards regulating the entities which are either engaged in manufacturing or contracting with medical devices in or out of the "blockchain ecosystem". This can be considered as one of the major steps towards the application of blockchain technology in the supply chain of the health sector [19]. However, it is to be seen how it influences the regulatory mechanism across the world and its efficacy in other parts of the world, where the socio-economic and socio-legal challenges are diverse from European nations.

13.3.1 Privacy Issues in Blockchain Technology

Almost all modern democracies have their existing privacy rights law. HIPAA[1] of USA is a strong example of this. In the USA, the existence of this Act would create legal challenges in the storage of data of "protected patient's information" on a public blockchain [14,15]. The situation is somewhat different in India as the regulation of medical data is not protected *per se* by any general or special legislation as it is in the USA but by interpretation and construction of various laws relating to medical data privacy [6,7]. Things could be far similar to the USA, once the proposed Personal Data Protection Bill is enacted in India.

As discussed, the primary challenge in including blockchain technology in the healthcare sector is privacy.

13.3.1.1 Privacy and Data Protection

The terms Privacy and Data protection are often used interchangeable and meant identical. However, there are substantial differences between the two with the former broader in the periphery than the latter, which exists primarily within the "world wide web" (www).

The essential requirement of privacy, as well as data protection, is the non-availability of personal data in the public domain on one hand and substantial managing power of the same (controlling) on the other hand. However, due to various reasons, much private information including name, date of birth, contact details, profession, etc. are readily available with various institutions, both public and private (online and offline). Data privacy laws are primarily intended to regulate the "information gathered" from being misused or transferred to interested parties for commercial purposes [4,7]. Adoption of "privacy laws" implies the incorporation of technical, administrative or physical measures to prevent such wrongs.

In India, majority of the rural and semi-urban populace are poverty-stricken. Government agencies lack minimum infrastructure for primary healthcare, and the challenge is multiplying with the increasing population density. In such strenuous circumstances, practical measures to restrain the violation of privacy may seem a luxury rather than a necessity unless a case of a breach bubbles up to visibility.

Privacy, however, is a fundamental right in India, of course, for them who choose to enforce it that way. Those who would want to avail it that way. But "privacy right" *per se* is absent physically in Part III[2] of the Constitution but is notionally inherent therein specifically in Article 21, which reads as under,

> No person shall be deprived of his life or personal liberty except according to the procedure established by law.

From time and again, the term "life" has been interpreted in its wholesome meaning to include all those aspects of life that are essential to make a person's existence more meaningful and worth living.[3]

The Data Protection Act, 1984, which came into force in 1988 in England authorises some rights to the people. The Act enables any person to be informed of and also get a copy of any electronic record which includes his or her personal records or information, which is with any person. Access to Health Records Act, 1990, also enables access to health records to the patients [8,9]. The reports are also subjected to the consent of the concerned patients prior to it being shown to the insurers or employers.[4]

13.3.1.1.1   *The Laws Prevailing in India to Address Medical Data Privacy*

Medical data privacy issue requires the understanding of a set of independent laws unless the Personal Data Protection Bill, 2019, is enforced. Till then, the formal laws which relate to medical data privacy in India call for independent scrutiny.

The situation is somehow different in India in the absence of any such law. The recent amendment to the Information Technology Act, 2000,[5] in India has seen the incorporation of Sections 43A[6] and 72A,[7] which calls for compensation in case of misuse of personal data. It, however, does not authorise a person to know or to get a copy of electronic data which is in possession of any other person. Again, there is no limitation in storing or retaining such data in Indian law.[8] The National Commission held[9] that non-furnishing of medical records to the patient does not constitute medical negligence. It specifically identified the absence of any legal duty thereof invoked by law or convention or practice in this regard – the State Commission in Md. Aslam v. Ideal Nursing Home[10] highlighted this vacuum and made the necessary recommendation to incorporate laws in this regard.

13.3.1.1.2   *Information Technology Act, 2000 (IT Act)*

The IT Act[11]came up *inter alia* to legitimise online agreements and regulate certain online unlawful and illegal activities. Data privacy is also covered under this Act but is not distinctively medical data. Thus, the general rules apply for data privacy *ipso facto* applies to medical data privacy. Blockchain, being a species of technology, therefore falls within the domain of IT Act 2000.

Privacy rights on the web are protected by invoking a comprehensive jurisdiction incorporated in Section 1[12] and Section 75[13] of the enactment. The Act is also empowered with adequate powers to punish the perpetrator and impose a hectic fine on the wrongdoer. Chapter IX[14] and XI[15] are testimony to this claim. The Act addresses the protection of data from being intercepted, manipulated and misused.

As discussed earlier, the recent amendment to the Act incorporating Sections 43A and 72A did provide some relief against the misuse of personal data.

Privacy issues: It has been debated that the right to share data on the part of the patient vests upon the criteria of consent.

13.3.2.2   Privacy and Consent

The right to privacy may be waived, legally by consent through an agreement, expressed or implied.

Consent, *per se*, is a legal term and is very much a part of the commercial law domain where *consensus ad idem* (meeting of minds) is a *sine qua non*. The mandate has also been codified in the Indian Contract Act, 1872.

Let us deliberate upon an elementary yet cardinal aspect of consent. This would help to understand the bifurcation it has from reality. Do we read the privacy policy before agreeing to that? If we don't, we take in consent as a mere formality both in practice and in litigation!

Before analysing the most probable answer, it is essential to understand the concept legally. Consent plays a vital role in almost all areas of law. In the law of contract, the word *consensus ad idem* is generally used to signify consent. It means thinking of the same thing in the same sense. Thus, when the parties enter into an agreement and consents, they voluntarily bind themselves to oblige [12,13,16,17]. In Indian marital laws, consent is one of the *sine qua non* of a valid marriage.[16] Criminal laws in India also recognise consent as a valid exception to the offence of rape.[17]

Coming down to the obvious answer, the former US Federal Trade Commission Chairman, John Leibowitz also said, "In many cases, consumers don't notice, read, or understand the privacy policies"".[18]

13.3.2.3   The Concept of Illusory Consent!

Another short question, can we afford a hugely expensive iPhone to turn into a brick? If one does not consent, one would not be able to update the software on the mobile phone. Hence that makes a phone as expensive as the iPhone of no use. Thus, the question of the relevance of these consent opportunities arises for a reasonable answer.

The legal effect of shifting the liability is practically imposition of a burden upon the consumer. And this burden is quite significant, e.g., what happens when the hospital mandates the dependents of a critical patient to sign a form (give a consent) prior to an operation, actually results in consenting to such procedure on the patient. Needless to say, the consent referred to here is an illusory one.

13.3.2.4   Over-Riding Consent

In cases of criminals, research data of previously published work. Do the consumer laws allow "you can always ask the consumer if it is ok to defraud?" The company or organisation should act as a steward. You can do what we usually do with such data.

Redress! What happens when something goes wrong?

Consent at the inception! Prompting the user when the software requests permission to access the location?

Once we start agreeing, we keep on deciding on subsequent situations. It seems we are on a slippery slope where we tend to waive it altogether. Maybe, we depend on the existence of a rather elusive superior law to protect us in case of a violation.

13.3.2.5   The Position of Data Protection Law in India: Can the State Be Construed as the Modern Data Controller?

Data protection law in the form of legislation *per se* is still missing in India. However, a much-debated Bill,[19] which was arguably introduced as a defence to the Aadhar case by the Government of India to prevent the inclusion of the right of privacy as an integral part of Fundamental Rights as enshrined in Part III of the Indian Constitution, at the apex court of the country. Irrespective of the outcome of the case, the absence of specific legislation protecting privacy rights and data protection has made the position very vulnerable in many avenues. This prompted judicial activism[20] to come as a savior of the Indian people has its specific limitation which proper legislation could have quickly addressed. Thus, this void has left the pillar of data protection and privacy rights solely on the findings of the Aadhar judgement. In other words, the Puttuswamy[21] case has become the foundation of privacy jurisprudence in modern India. As the Supreme Court incorporated the right to privacy to be within the list of fundamental rights, the government fails to find an answer to balance the developing pressure of private players, who act as the backbone of growing Indian economy and the inherent right of the people of 130 crore people of India. Irrespective of the absence of specific legislation which is expected to have a blanket application over every aspect, India has a set of subject-specific legislation which incorporates the issue of privacy and data protection [18,19].

In the Aadhar case,[22] the state was considered to be the violator in chief. Surprisingly, the proposed Bill of 2018 and 2019 has noticeable loopholes which allow the government to claim protection in data violation cases. Another interesting move may be to move the state to the position of a data protection controller. In such a situation, the state would be in a quasi-judicial function. It may in the majority of cases be of help to ordinary people in protecting their right to privacy.

13.3.2   CREDIBILITY

Healthcare stands on the mere existence of credibility when it comes to the authenticity of any medical test or the outcome of a diagnosis. The majority of such records are credible information that is generated after complying with the due process established by law to which it is subjected to. The credibility of such records and data depends upon the mere existence of such date at source and not at the nodes. If, for instance, an USG of a pregnant lady is sought for in criminal investigation under the Medical Termination of Pregnancy Act,[23] it is more relevant to rely on the report generated by the testing agency rather than the accused or the victim in the case. In the case of the latter, the scope of challenge and verification is much broader than the former, which *inter alia* reduces the overall tenure of the litigation.

13.3.3   REGULATION

The process of regulating maintenance, storage and retention of medical data is far and few. It is rarer when it comes to managing the said data electronically. The mobility of such data in the absence of regulation becomes volatile when it comes to its credibility, reliability and admissibility in the court of law. Here, blockchain may play a dynamic role in meeting the requisite regulatory challenges of authenticity and credibility. The regulations would also play a positive role in eliminating the flaws and loopholes in the blockchain mechanism to make it more acceptable and admissible.

13.3.4   DECENTRALISATION

Blockchain technology gets its potential strength from its decentralised approach. The users in a decentralised system are free to control the data, and once the technology makes it incorrigible, the said data gets the required authenticity law demands. Absence of a centralised agency in this regard carries with it a host of benefits like brushing aside high-handedness, tampering of data, corruption and other limitations of a centralised system.

13.4   VIABILITY OF BLOCKCHAIN TECHNOLOGY

Blockchain technology can do wonders once it is applied in the healthcare sector strategically. The conventional methods of recording and storing data are not only difficult to maintain but impractical in the modern world to regulate upon. To explain this position, a case analysis is given below, which elaborates on the challenges of data collection, storing and regulating the sale of certain prohibited drugs.

13.4.1   REGULATORY DIRECTIVES TO COLLECT DATA
OF PATIENTS (IN INDIA): A CASE STUDY

The situation is not very encouraging in case of data management of medicines sold in the pharmacy sector in India. There are certain drugs and medications which are prohibited from being sold without a proper prescription from an authorised doctor. While prescribing certain scheduled medicines, the doctors also need to be very careful of the consequences of such medications. Consequences thereof, both positive and negative, need to be made clear to the respective patient.

There are specific laws that regulate the functioning of medicine and pharmacy stores. Only specific pharmacy is permitted to sell certain drugs. A special license is required to be acquired to authorise the sale or distribution of those drugs. The law directs those licensed dealers and stores to make and retain a copy of the prescription before the selling of those scheduled medications to the patient. The reason for such a direction is to keep track of those scheduled medicines. The periodic external audit is also done in these stores to keep a check on unauthorised selling of such medications and drugs.

Apart from this, there is an element of discretion in case the pharmacist is confused or unsure about the integrity of the drugs prescribed. He may also make a copy of the same securing the safety of the patient. Inclusion of blockchain technology may easily control this complicated process and assist enormously in identifying the patients and the number of medicines sold within a specific period.

Absence of proper regulatory mechanism or introduction of technology in the healthcare sector has seen an unprecedented collection of personal data for specific economic reasons. The prescriptions are scanned nowadays by many medical stores and pharmacists to study, inter alia, the flow of medicines in a particular area. This helps them to keep a track on the sequence of medications. In recent years, medication for a prolonged period to combat chronic diseases like asthma, high blood pressure or diabetes is prescribed. The flooding of new medicine in the market, coupled with the pressure on the doctors to prescribe them, may be to keep the pharmaceutical industry flooding with profits. The situation is tragic at times that even when medicine for high blood pressure is mistakenly given to a person, the medication needs to be continued for his lifetime.

Other exciting development in the absence of proper regulatory framework includes sharing of medical data across networks promoting telemarketing, developing an informal relationship with the patients and alluring them with freebies like unique benefit cards (where points would be added which can later be redeemed). In the garb of such allurement, the data of the users are stored, studied and used to regulate pharma industry [9,14,15].

A little up the hierarchy are organisations like Yellow Pages and Just Dial. They have their apps online on both android and mac platforms. On a grass root level, however, they generally approach the smaller organisations and pharmacy stores. To be within Just Dial, i.e., whenever one searches for medicines through this app, registered medicine stores are referred with contact details. Their standard marketing policy includes home delivery facilities, in case the store does not have any home delivery facilities, to individually tie up with home delivery business units like Swiggy and Zomato to deliver the medicine ordered. In this way, all the medication ordered by customers (patients) is recorded and stored for various reasons. It is not the amount of medicine that an end-user spends per month, but the medication *per se*, they are consuming periodically is recorded. This colossal data that gathered after a couple of years enables the organisations to sell the said data to a third party. On the occasion of a company being sold or merged with another company, the entire medical records, including the medicinal habits of people, are now owned by a new organisation that the end customers never knew or anticipated.

13.4.2 The Change in the Making

Systematic application of blockchain technology in healthcare industry can effectively mitigate some of the significant risks pertaining to inconsistencies in the patient medical record, vulnerability of data in the hand of prospective perpetrators and problems in retrieving medical records on demand [20].

Tech professions globally believe that blockchain technology has the potential to streamline healthcare data. Significant challenges [21,22,23] in medical record management like recording, storing and accessing data securely; protection of sensitive medical records; autonomy to the patients over such data. However, to revolutionise this industry, a custom-built healthcare blockchain is still to be developed and constructed.

Blockchain is quite different from the existing technologies available and used to keep medical records and related data in healthcare. However, it must be noted that the main difference lies in the application of technology. Identifying the viability of the technology is dependent on the law to a great extent, as the current blockchain technology is contradicting the data privacy laws in many ways [24,25].

13.4.3 Example of Incentive to Promote Blockchain

One of the examples of incentivising the practice of blockchain can be found in the practice of MedRec,[24] which incentivise the miners. They are mostly the researchers in medicine and professionals involved in healthcare. They are provided with benefits like aggregated data accessibility and other records retrieved and shared with the consent of the patient for epidemiological studies [10,11].

13.4.4 How it Is Better Than Conventional (Traditional) Methods?

The conventional method generally focused on disease detection, where many patients with various ailments wait to be diagnosed by the doctor. The doctor, in such manner of practice, seldom relies on the previous medical conditions or reports. The patients too were serious about preserving their medical records after they are free from such physical challenges – shorter the time is taken to recover briefer the preservation of the medical history [12,13].

In many jurisdictions, traditional practitioners exercise their business unlawfully. Absence of state control over such practitioners leads to tax evasion in a majority of the cases. This leads to a substantial economic loss of the state and consequently to the development of the country. Many tax raids on successful medical professionals have revealed similar outcomes.[25]

Another interesting challenge is the privacy of the patient. In many cases, the discussion between the doctor and the patient is done in the presence of other patients. Even the physical integrity of the patient is jeopardised with the majority of the physical tests are conducted on the patient in the presence of outsiders.

Traditional practice generally involves disease centric approach and does not work well in cases of comorbidity.[26]

TABLE 13.2

Contrasting Traditional and Modern Method of Medical Practice (Legal Perspectives)

Sl. No.	Traditional Method	Modern Method
1	Chance of irregular, unlawful and illegality practices are higher	Since everything is transparent, change of illegality, illegal & inconsistent practices are less
2	Tax evasion is rampant	Tax and other regulatory payments are identifiable, and hence tax evasion is easily avoided
3	Patients' privacy depends upon the will of the practitioner	Practitioners are well aware of their responsibilities, including protecting the privacy of the patient. However, a customised way of using blockchain is necessary to make it HIPAA (and other regulations across the world) compliant
4	Retention of medical records after some time becomes challenging for most of the patients. Hence, the subsequent treatment methods become experimental	Chance of losing data is minimal in this process, making the treatment less experimental and patient-centric
5	Referring the patient to other doctors with a specialisation is negligible	Patients are referred to other doctors (in case of complications in other health areas) for a comprehensive treatment of the patient
6	The position of elderly patients with many complications are vulnerable to wrong treatment	Change of such negligence is reduced comprehensively
7	The doctors have little alternative but to refer the patients for multiple pathological tests	This is easily avoided because of the availability of the previous record, helping to reduce the expenses and time for treatment
8	Proper connectivity between the medical practitioner and the policymaker is missing	A systematic representation of the trending medical challenges is automatically sent to the policymakers (Government) to take adequate measures to control a subsequent pandemic etc. immediately

Most private hospitals evade tax: CAG, The Hindu, available at, https://www.thehindu.com/news/national/most-private-hospitals-evade-tax-cag/article19380559.ece.

Traditional practitioners can exercise their business illegally, without control by the state, and may fail to pay state taxes. They can violate patients' privacy, jeopardise patients' physical integrity and fail to provide patients with information on a treatment's side effects. Traditional practitioners may fail to refer patients, who would benefit from effective therapies (e.g. those with tuberculosis or HIV), to conventional medical services [26]. Also, if they fail to collect information on diseases they observe or transmit this information to healthcare authorities, they jeopardise the quality of health information systems.[27]

A brief set of differences between the two are given in Table 13.2.[28]

13.5   CONCLUSION AND RECOMMENDATION

Significant changes in the domain of healthcare can be made for the better with the formulation of new laws and changes in the existing laws and regulations prevailing in our country. Incorporation of technology in medical data management can go a long way in multifaceted protection of stakeholders. The new Data Protection Bill is a welcome step forward in this direction. However, there are technology-specific challenges involved in blockchain technology as being faced in HIPAA. Evolution of this new technology mitigating the challenges brought forth, primarily by privacy issues, needs to be addressed as well.

Once that is done, there would be a revolution in the healthcare sector in the decades to come.

Blockchain technology is capable of mitigating challenges that was literally impossible to address before its existence. The beneficiaries include inter alia, the patient and the health of the patient. It assists the healthcare assistants to understand what medication is best for the patient and eliminates confusion about previous medical conditions of each specific patient. A lot of litigation pertaining to medical negligence can be reduced dramatically with the transparency in the system. Availability of data on demand to those requiring the same can save a lot of time and unnecessary delay in medication. This will revolutionize the way healthcare industry functions for good.

Formally, blockchain technology as it stands today cannot be adopted, irrespective of the multiple benefits it brings with it. Because of the existing significant limitations in the realm of law, it would be challenging to be formally accepted. Thus, the technology requires adapting to fit within the legal framework of specific jurisdictions. While developing the change, technology must focus on challenges of privacy issues. Similarly, the traditional systems to avail the benefits blockchain technology could bring to the healthcare sector must make room for it as well, once the mandatory challenges are addressed by making necessary changes in the technology. A network of technical and legal experts must work in tandem to make the technology legally enabled. This interdisciplinary research would help to revolutionise healthcare sector for the years to come and make it more patient-centric.

NOTES

1   The Health Insurance Portability and Accountability Act of 1996.
2   Fundamental Rights, Part III of the Constitution of India, 1950.
3   Olga Tellis and Ors. V. Bombay Municipal Corporation and Ors, 1985.
4   Access to Medical Records Act, 1988.
5   Ins. by Section 22 of Act 10 of 2009, (w.e.f. 27-10-2009).
6   Ibid.

7 Ibid.
8 NCDRC 1995 (1) CPJ 232: 1995 (1) CPR 661 (NCDRC) 1996 CCJ 70.
9 Poona Medical Foundation Ruby Hall Clinic v. Marutirao L. Titkare.
10 Orissa SCDRC 1994 (1) CPR 619.
11 Act No. 21 of 2000.
12 Ibid.
13 Ibid.
14 Ibid.
15 Ibid.
16 Section 4 of Special Marriage Act, 1954 and Section 5 of Hindu Marriage Act, 1955.
17 Section 375 Indian Penal Code, 1860.
18 How 'Do Not Track' Ended Up Going Nowhere, available at https://www.vox.com/2016/1/4/11588418/how-do-not-track-ended-up-going-nowhere accessed on April 9th 2020.
19 The Personal Data Protection Bill, 2019.
20 Civil Liberties v. Union of India ((1997) 1 SCC 301) commonly known as the Telephone tapping case is also one of the leading cases concerning data privacy in India.
21 Justice K. S. Puttuswamy (Retd.) and Anr. vs Union of India and Ors.
22 Ibid.
23 Act 34 of 1971.
24 Ariel Ekblaw and Asaf Azaria, *MedRec: Medical Data Management on the Blockchain,* available at https://viral.media.mit.edu/pub/medrec/release/1.
25 Most private hospitals evade tax: CAG, The Hindu, available at, https://www.thehindu.com/news/national/most-private-hospitals-evade-tax-cag/article19380559.ece.
26 Traditional and Modern Medicine Harmonizing the Two Approaches: A Report of the Consultation Meeting on Traditional and Modern Medicine: Harmonizing the Two Approaches, 22-26 November 1999, Beijing, China, available at https://www.evidence-based.net/files/trad&mod_med.pdf.
27 Don Tapscott and Alex Tapscott, *What Blockchain Could Mean for Your Health Data,* available at, https://hbr.org/2020/06/what-blockchain-could-mean-for-your-health-data.
28 Ibid.

REFERENCES

1. Abouelmehdi K., Beni-Hessane A., and Khaloufi H. 2018. Big healthcare data: Preserving security and privacy. *Journal of Big Data* 5, 1.
2. Barrows R.C., and Clayton P.D. 1996. Privacy, confidentiality, and electronic medical records. *Journal of the American Medical Informatics Association* 3(2), 139–148.
3. Bellazzi R. 2014. Big data and biomedical informatics: A challenging opportunity. *Yearbook of Medical Informatics*, 9(1), 8–13.
4. Borry P., Bentzen B.H., Budin-Ljøsne I., et al. 2018. The challenges of the expanded availability of genomic information: An agenda-setting paper. *Journal of Community Genetics*, 9(2), 103–116.
5. Coos A. 2018. EU vs US: How Do Their Data Privacy Regulations Square Off?https://www.endpointprotector.com/blog/eu-vs-us-how-do-their-data-protection-regulations-square-off/.
6. Dove E.S., and Phillips M. 2015. Privacy law, data sharing policies, and medical data: A comparative perspective. In Gkoulalas-Divanis A. and Loukides, G. (Eds) *Medical Data Privacy Handbook*, pp.639–678.Springer, Cham.
7. Ghidini G. 2006. Intellectual property and competition law. https://epdf.pub/intellectual-property-and-competition-law-the-innovation-nexus.html.

8. Green, A. 2020. Complete guide to privacy laws in the US. https://www.varonis.com/blog/us-privacy-laws/.

9. Gkoulalas-Divanis A., and Loukides G. (Eds.). 2015. *Medical Data Privacy Handbook.* Springer, Cham.

10. Haas S., Wohlgemuth S., Echizen I., Sonehara N., and Müller G. 2011. Aspects of privacy for electronic health records. *International Journal of Medical Informatics*, 80(2), e26–e31.

11. Karegar F., Gerber N., Volkamer M., and Fischer-Hübner S. 2018. Helping john to make informed decisions on using social login. Proceedings of the 33rd Annual ACM Symposium on Applied Computing, pp. 1165–1174.

12. Kobie N. 2019. The Complicated Truth about China's Social Credit System. https://www.wired.co.uk/article/china-social-credit-system-explained.

13. Malin B.A. 2005. An evaluation of the current state of genomic data privacy protection technology and a roadmap for the future. *Journal of the American Medical Informatics Association*, 12(1), 28–34.

14. Pernot-Leplay E. 2020. Data Privacy Law in China: Comparison with the EU and U.S. Approaches. https://pernot-leplay.com/data-privacy-law-china-comparison-europe-usa/.

15. Price W.N. and Cohen I.G. 2019. Privacy in the age of medical big data. *Nature Medicine*, 25(1), 37–43.

16. Vora J., Italiya P., Tanwar S., Tyagi S., Kumar N., Obaidat M.S., and Hsiao K.F. 2018. Ensuring privacy and security in E-health records. In 2018 International Conference on Computer, Information and Telecommunication Systems (CITS), France, (pp. 1–5). IEEE.

17. Walters R. 2018. China and US Compete To Dominate Big Data. https://www.ft.com/content/e33a6994-447e-11e8-93cf-67ac3a6482fd.

18. Health Europa. 2020. Blockchain in Healthcare. Retrieved May 25, 2021, from HIMSS: https://www.himss.org/resources/blockchain-healthcare

19. HIMSS. n.d. Blockchain: the Trust Solution for the Healthcare Industry? (2020, January 23). Retrieved May 25, 2021, from Health Europa: https://www.healtheuropa.eu/blockchain-the-trust-solution-for-healthcare/96840/.

20. Wetzels M., Broers E., Peters P., Feijs L., Widdershoven J., and Habibovic M. 2018. Patient perspectives on health data privacy and management: "Where is my data and whose is it?" *International Journal of Telemedicine and Applications*, 2018, 3838747. https://doi.org/10.1155/2018/3838747

21. WTO. Agreement on Trade Related Aspects of Intellectual Property. https://www.wto.org/english/docs_e/legal_e/27-trips.pdf.

22. Wong R. 2012. Big data privacy. *Journal of Information Technology Software Engineering*, 2(5), 114.

23. Wright A. 2017. 8 Things You Need to Know about India's Economy. https://www.weforum.org/agenda/2017/10/eight-key-facts-about-indias-economy-in-2017.

24. U.S.-EU Safe Harbor Framework. https://www.ftc.gov/tips-advice/business-center/privacy-and-security/u.s.-eu-safe-harbor-framework.

25. Madhok A.K. vs Centre for Fingerprinting & Diagnostics (CDFD). 2007, Decision_26102007_06 (RTI Commissioner 2007).

26. Mr. Surupsingh Hrya Naik vs State Of Maharashtra, AIR 2007 Bom 121 (Bombay High Court March 23, 2007).

Index